The Man TURNED BLUE

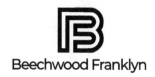

Beechwood Franklyn

Published in the UK in 2022 by Beechwood Franklyn

Paperback ISBN 978-1-8384949-2-6
eBook ISBN 978-1-8384949-3-3

Cover design and typeset by SpiffingCovers.com

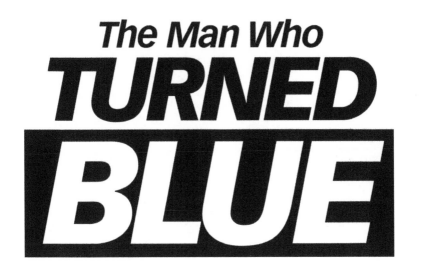

The Man Who TURNED BLUE

Dr Barry Monk

Contents

FOREWORD

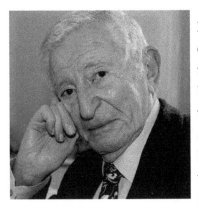

I was honoured to be invited, once again, by Dr Barry Monk, to write a foreword to his new book, having quite recently, written one for his 'Lifeline', a collection of essays on the National Health Service, which I was delighted to read had won the 2022 BMA medical book award in the category 'Good Medical Practice'.

This present volume is a collection of interesting dermatological cases. I have to confess that dermatology was not taken very seriously when I was a medical student at the old Radcliffe Infirmary in Oxford. In 1947 the course entailed attendance at the weekly outpatient skin clinic for three months. Our consultant was Dr Alice Carleton, a middle-aged lady of quite striking appearance as she had her white hair dyed an attractive blue.

We inspected, with her, a stream of patients, and long names were attributed to their various conditions. Treatment seemed to be the application of a variety of peculiar preparations designed to make dry conditions moist and wet conditions dry.

We were reassured that dermatological conditions never appeared in our final examinations. I hang my head in shame when I allowed this fact to influence thetime I allowed for my study of skin diseases.

Dr Barry Monk, who I am proud to say is a nephew of mine, has brought together a fascinating collection of patients who presented to him as a dermatologist where meticulous clinical care, in what reminds me of a Sherlock Holmes approach to diagnosis will often result in a successful outcome for the patient. I am sure that readers of this fascinating book will come to regard dermatology (and dermatologists) in a new light.

Professor Harold Ellis, CBE, FRCS,

Emeritus Professor of Anatomy, Guy's Hospital, London

November 2022

CHAPTER ONE

GOING LIKE A BOMB[1]

A gentleman came into my private consulting room and sat down rather diffidently, facing me across my desk. He was in his mid-seventies and smartly turned out in the usual style of a member of the local gentry, well-polished brown brogue shoes, crushed-strawberry corduroy trousers, tweed jacket, checked shirt and tie. From the look on his face, he was obviously troubled, and I invited him to tell me all.

He explained that some three months previously he had broken out in a most distressing, itchy rash, which was keeping him awake at night and pre-occupying him every hour of the day. He was otherwise healthy, took no medications, had no allergies, and led a generally blameless life. He was at a loss to explain what had afflicted him and was afraid that his visits to his excellent local GP had given him no explanation or relief. He admitted that he was beside himself with worry about it.

I invited him to undress so that I could examine his skin. The problem was immediately apparent. Over the back, buttocks and limbs there were numerous, randomly distributed

---

1 By a curious coincidence, Chapter 1 of my first book, LIFELINE, is also titled 'Going Like A Bomb'. The subject matter is totally different, but once again, it seemed just right.

lesions, all rather uniform in appearance and about the size of a fifty pence piece. Each was a vivid red colour with a slightly crusted oozy surface. I could see why he was so alarmed.

I reassured him that I was confident that I would be able to assist him, and asked him to get dressed. I explained that the appearance was absolutely characteristic of a rather curious condition called discoid eczema[2].

Discoid eczema is a puzzling disorder, but a diagnosis which I always enjoy making as it improves so dramatically with treatment. Typically, patients are most commonly men in the middle years of life. There is often no antecedent history of eczema, until the totally abrupt onset of the rash, which is associated with severe and relentless itching and often an associated frenzy of scratching. The bedclothes and pyjamas are often reported to be covered in blood.

Almost invariably the condition is provoked by stress, and if the patient is stressed before the onset of the rash, it goes without saying that being awake all night with a relentlessly itchy rash does not help their situation.

I explained the diagnosis and its likely cause to my patient. I advised that the use of a potent topical steroid cream at night associated with a sedative to ensure a proper night's sleep almost invariably resolved matters, as long as whatever was stressing him could also be resolved. But this is often

---

2   'Discoid' means 'coin shaped'; in the original description of the condition by a French dermatologist in 1854, the lesions were described as all being the size of a five-franc coin.

the real problem; we all talk about stress, but no one really understands what stress is, and why in some people it provokes such a dramatic rash. I wondered to myself what on earth was stressing this man who appeared to lead a quiet and comfortable life, yet others who seem to lead lives of relentless pressure appear to thrive on it.

"Oh, Dr Monk", he said woefully, "you just can't imagine what stress I am under", and he proceeded to tell me his story. He lived in solitary splendour in the house where he had been born; it is a magnificent building, one of the finest homes in the county and full of treasures. The house had originally been built in the nineteenth century by his grandfather who had been one of the foremost architects of the Victorian period. In fact, an acquaintance of mine, who lives nearby, told me that he remembers, as a small boy, going to the house each week with his father, a clock repairer, whose job it was to wind the forty-six clocks in the house. Electricity had only been installed after the Second World War.

My patient had spent several fruitless years attempting to give the property to a major national charity. They had been very keen to have it, along with its contents, but only if he would undertake to give them £1 million as well[3], something to which he had been reluctant to agree. It turned out that he had now, at last, found a buyer for his house, and was finally in the process of planning his move.

---

3   I hadn't appreciated that it is quite routine for charities to expect a 'dowry' to accompany such gifts.

"Had he," I asked him, "come across anything unexpected when clearing a lifetime of possessions?". I suggested, a little playfully, "perhaps a long-forgotten birthday card from an old aunt with a ten-shilling postal order inside it or a school exercise book with geography homework that he might have been in trouble for not handing in".

He looked at me, for a few seconds, and then said, "Well there was something, and that's where the trouble really started." It's at moments like this when I am most grateful that I am not a GP, expected to cure all the ills of the world in ten minutes. In private practice, I have longer consultation slots, but more to the point, I am my own master, and if I choose to let the patient talk, that's my prerogative. On this occasion, I made the right decision.

He explained that amongst the endless items that he had sorted through, he had come across a curious brass cylinder, about ten inches in length, with a long pink ribbon emerging from its end. He had inspected it carefully but couldn't imagine what it was, although having lived his entire life in a house crammed with works of art, he knew there was 'something about it'. He placed it on the kitchen table and carried on with the treasure hunt.

A few days later, an old friend had popped in for a cup of tea. As he sat down, he suddenly announced, "Good God, what are you doing with that thing?", pointing to the mystery object. "Don't you know what it is?"

My patient explained that he had no idea what it was, and that was exactly why it was on the table. His companion explained that it was a First World War hand grenade, of a type used by the Royal Flying Corps. It would be thrown out of an aeroplane, with the pilot keeping hold of the ribbon, which would trigger the detonator[4].

"We must call the police at once", said my patient, to which his friend replied, "Oh, no. We can't do that; you would be in the most terrible trouble for having a bomb without proper authority."

My patient had led a calm and gentle life and wasn't used to this sort of excitement, but eventually, they hatched a plan.

---

4   These were officially known as the British Hand Grenade No2. The hand grenade had been quite an innovation in World War One, having been first used in the Mexican Revolution of 1907.

The British War Office and several foreign countries have placed large orders with Mr F. Marten Hale, of the Cotton Powder Company, Ltd., for his new bomb designed for dropping from aeroplanes or airships. Important tests were carried out two or three days ago at Eastchurch, and the experts expressed themselves as surprised at the results. The features of the bomb are that, dropped at any angle or position and at any speed that the airship may be travelling at, the projectile will almost immediately regain and maintain its vertical position in descent, so that it hits its target perfectly plumb and nose downwards, the tendency to somersaults and wobbling which is so apparent in all other bombs entirely disappearing.

The bomb is so sensitive that it will explode on the slightest retardation due to impact, even on water, soft ground, mud, or snow. The tests were made on a Short biplane piloted by Flying-master F. B. Parker, R.N. Lieutenant Pierse, R.N., seated behind, manipulated the bombs. The "Hale" bomb, it is claimed, will pierce 3in of steel armor plate, and will be equally effective on sloping sides as on a flat surface. Should it hit a fortress gun it would smash it, and if the bomb fell a few yards away it would make such a displacement of the earth as to upset the foundation of the gun and put it out of action. Mr Hale is the inventor of numerous explosive designs used by Britain and other countries. One of the latest was an illuminating grenade fired from rifles for use in night attacks.

Figure 1: From the Wallace County Chronicle, Kansas, USA

They waited until it was dark, and then went out into the rather large garden, found a discreet spot well away from the house, and dug a hole in which they buried the object, marking its place with a flag. My patient's friend assured him that he had 'an old army pal' who would know what to do, and true to his word, a few nights later he reappeared in the company of another elderly gentleman, who some sixty years previously had had some experience of handling ordnance.

As he described it, I could picture the scene like something of an upmarket version of *Last of the Summer Wine.* The three intrepid heroes had ventured back into the garden and by torchlight had located the flag and retrieved the grenade, which by some miracle they had then managed to make safe without mishap.

My patient looked at me with a languid expression, "So, now you know why I am stressed, Dr Monk."

I reassured him that all would be well with his skin, handed him his prescription, and asked him to return in a few weeks so that I could check on his progress.

In due course, he came back to the clinic, and I was delighted to see that the rash was resolved and he now was free of his tormenting itching. "How was the house move going?" I ventured.

"Oh, it's very difficult," he explained. "I am trying to pack up the library. I have got ten thousand books and only room for two thousand in the new house."

Discoid eczema remains one of the most enigmatic conditions which I see as a dermatologist and one of the most satisfying to treat. And stress can manifest itself in a myriad of ways.

CHAPTER TWO

AN OLD-FASHIONED DIAGNOSIS

There are few things that I enjoy more as a dermatologist than when I am asked to see a patient who is baffling my medical colleagues. One Tuesday morning, I was in my clinic, trying to work my way through a long list of patients and already running late, when the telephone rang. It was the sister on one of the acute medical wards at the hospital. They had a patient on the ward who was obviously unwell, but no one could quite work out what was the diagnosis and the consultant would be keen to have my opinion.

"Of course," I replied, "Send him straight down and I will see him".

Sometime later, the gentleman in question arrived. He was in his early sixties, but looked older, and was obviously frail and unwell. He had arrived at my clinic in a wheelchair, being unable to stand unaided. He had been admitted a few days earlier with a story of weight loss and anaemia and with severe pain in his bones. From that history, there had been a strong suspicion that he had some form of cancer, but extensive investigation had been unrevealing.

With some difficulty, we managed to help him onto the examination couch. He was thin and gaunt and somewhat unkempt. His teeth were in poor shape with swollen and bleeding gums. His skin showed extensive areas of bruising, and with careful examination with a magnifying glass, there were also numerous little areas of bleeding into the skin around the hair follicles on the limbs and trunk. As I continued to look at the skin, the diagnosis began to dawn on me, and I was able to identify a physical sign which I had read about but never actually seen; the hairs on the body were very short and oddly shaped, and described in older textbooks as 'cork-screw' hairs. This was a case of scurvy.

Scurvy is a condition which is caused by a dietary deficiency of ascorbic acid (Vitamin C). It has a long history, having been particularly prevalent in seafarers in the days of sailing ships. In the seventeenth and eighteenth centuries, scurvy had been a major cause of death and debility in sailors on long voyages. In those days, there was no system for preserving food on board, and in the Royal Navy, the sailors survived largely on a diet of salted beef, ships' biscuits and rum.

Scurvy usually appeared among the sailors after a few weeks at sea. Typically, it began with swollen, bleeding gums, painful limbs, (due to bleeding into the bone), bruising and ulceration of the skin, with poor wound healing and festering wounds associated with extreme lethargy and exhaustion and ultimately death. There are documented cases in which as many as fifty percent or more of a ship's company died of scurvy in the course of a long voyage, and it was certainly a greater hazard to the crew than the risk of shipwreck or gunfire from enemy ships.

There were endless theories as to the cause of scurvy, and it had been observed that sailors who supplemented their diet by catching and eating ships' rats appeared immune[5].

James Lind was the naval surgeon who finally established the role of citrus fruits in the prevention and treatment of scurvy among seafarers. Lind was born in Edinburgh in 1716 to a merchant family. He studied medicine in Edinburgh but left without formal qualifications to become an apprentice surgeon in the Royal Navy. He saw service in the West Indies and off the coast of West Africa, and like every medical officer of the time would have seen numerous cases of scurvy. Lind's interest in the subject was further stimulated by reports of George Anson's four-year circumnavigation of the globe, in which it was reported that over half the crew had died of scurvy.

In 1747, Lind was appointed ship's surgeon on HMS Salisbury, one of the Royal Navy's newest vessels, which put to sea with the objective of effecting a blockade of the Spanish fleet in the Bay of Biscay. As Salisbury's time at sea continued, cases of scurvy began to emerge, and Lind designed a clinical experiment, which has come to be regarded as the first controlled clinical trial in medical history.

---

5   It is now known that unlike many animals, rats synthesise their own Vitamin C

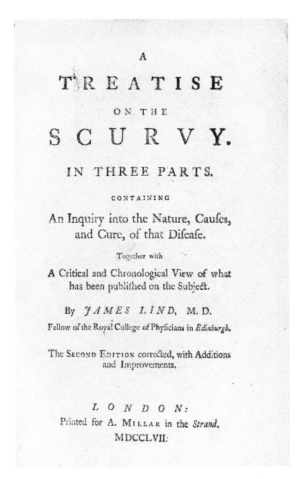

A

T R E A T I S E

ON THE

S C U R V Y.

IN THREE PARTS,

CONTAINING

An Inquiry into the Nature, Caufes,
and Cure, of that Difeafe.

Together with

A Critical and Chronological View of what
has been publifhed on the Subject.

By *JAMES LIND*, M. D.

Fellow of the Royal College of Phyficians in *Edinburgh*,

The SECOND EDITION corrected, with Additions
and Improvements,

L O N D O N:
Printed for A. MILLAR in the *Strand*,
MDCCLVII.

Figure 2: James Lind's classic work on scurvy (1757).

He took twelve affected sailors and divided them into six pairs.
Each pair, in addition to their normal food ration, was given
something which had been claimed, without much evidence,
to cure scurvy. One pair was given a quart of cider daily,
one was given twenty-five drops of elixir of vitriol (sulphuric
acid), one pair six spoonfuls of vinegar, one had half a pint of
seawater daily, one received two oranges and a lemon daily,
and the last group a spicy paste and a drink of barley water.

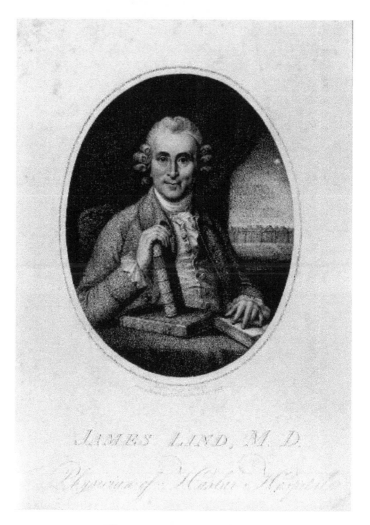

Figure 3: Dr James Lind MD,
(by permission of the Wellcome Collection)

Within a week, the pair who had a daily ration of oranges and a lemon was dramatically improved to the extent that they were fit to resume their normal duties. All of the others had continued to deteriorate.

Lind left the navy the following year and returned to Edinburgh to complete his medical studies. In 1753 he published *A Treatise on Scurvy* including an account of his experiment. The Admiralty, ever mindful of the cost implications, were doubtful about implementing Lind's recommendation that every sailor should be given a daily ration of lemon juice, but ships' captains, who had seen the dreadful impact of the disease, soon began to arrange for their crews to be supplied with fresh fruit on board ship. Captain Cook was an early enthusiast for Lind's ideas and arranged that on his three great voyages of exploration to the Pacific,[6] his crew were provided with pickled cabbage, which we now know also contains Vitamin C, supplemented wherever possible by fresh fruit. It is said that none of his crew developed scurvy.

It was only in 1790 that the Admiralty finally relented and ordered that every sailor was to have a daily ration of the juice of a lemon added to his rum ration, a useful method of ensuring compliance[7], but by this time, scurvy had already been effectively eliminated. Curiously, other countries were sceptical of this British innovation, which ensured that the Royal Navy was able to dominate the high seas for nearly two hundred years.[8]

---

6   On his first voyage, Cook discovered New Zealand and Australia, but the original purpose of the expedition was to make observations from the Pacific of the transit of Venus, a phenomenon which only occurs approximately every eighty years.

7   Lemon juice was replaced with lime juice in 1860, as limes were cheaper. Subsequently, sailors in the Royal Navy came to be nicknamed 'Limeys' by their American counterparts.

8   The other factor which ensured British naval supremacy was the chronometer designed and built by John Harrison, which was the first instrument to allow accurate measurement of time at sea, which in turn allowed the reliable calculation of longitude, essential for navigation.

Lind returned to naval service as the commanding officer of the Royal Naval Hospital Haslar in Gosport. He conducted important research into the transmission of typhus[9] and invented a system for desalinating sea water. He died in 1794. It was to be over a hundred years (in the early 1900s) before ascorbic acid, Vitamin C, was identified as the active ingredient in citrus fruits and green vegetables that prevents scurvy. It is now known that ascorbic acid plays an essential role in the synthesis of collagen, and hence deficiency is associated with fragility of the skin and poor wound healing.

So, how had my patient come to develop scurvy? Bedford is about as far from the sea as you can get in the United Kingdom, and he had never been a seafarer. I asked him about his diet and he looked a little sheepish. He eventually admitted that he didn't eat any solid food at all, his entire calorie intake being provided by extra strength lager, two cans for breakfast, two for lunch and two for tea. I explained the diagnosis to him and arranged for him to be provided with some Vitamin C tablets from the pharmacy as well as a daily orange from the catering department, and when I visited him on the ward a few days later his condition was dramatically improved.

Of course, if he had lived entirely on gin and tonic rather than lager, he wouldn't have had a problem at all, because the slice of lemon in the gin would have protected him. However, I wouldn't recommend anyone living on gin and tonic either; you might not get scurvy, but you would soon become

---

9   Typhus is a group of infectious diseases caused by rickettsial bacteria, usually spread by lice or fleas and occurring in epidemics, more commonly in conditions of overcrowding or privation.

deficient in Vitamin B1 and B2, and end up with pellagra and beri beri.

It is remarkable to think that over two hundred years after James Lind's observations, we still see scurvy from time to time, most often in people, occasionally children, who have adopted a very restrictive or faddish diet, deficient in Vitamin C. It is always a rewarding diagnosis to make.

CHAPTER THREE

THE MAN WHO TURNED BLUE

As a dermatologist, I am well aware that we are often perceived, unfairly of course, as mainly dealing with trivial medical conditions. Indeed, I suspect that some of my colleagues in other specialities don't think that we are really 'proper doctors' at all. So, it is all the more gratifying when a problem comes along which really allows us to show our worth.

One Monday morning I was parking my car in the hospital car park, when one of my colleagues, a consultant cardiologist, came rushing up to me in a state of some excitement.

"Thank goodness you're here, Barry," he greeted me, "We need you to come and see a patient on the ward."

I never refuse an invitation like that, and as we set off towards the long corridor which runs the length of the hospital, I asked him to tell me about the case.

"He's a twenty-year-old chap who was admitted as an emergency last night, having gone blue at home," he explained.

I stopped and looked at him. "Well, that sounds much more your field than mine", I replied.

"No, we've done all the usual tests, chest X-ray, ECG, blood gases and the like, and everything is normal. And to make things worse, his dad is an ambulance paramedic, and furious that we don't seem to know what to do".

It was certainly a puzzle, and as we walked on, my brain was frantically sorting through the diagnostic possibilities. We arrived at the ward to be greeted by a remarkable sight. The patient was sitting up in bed. His mother sat by his bedside, quietly weeping, and his father stood facing her, his arms crossed and with a look of thunder on his face. Around the bed was a large cluster of junior doctors, medical students, nurses and health care assistants, all apparently waiting for me.

Suddenly, I was hit by a flash of inspiration like an Old Testament prophet, and as I approached the patient's bedside, I whispered something to the ward sister, carefully making sure that no one else had heard me. I introduced myself to the patient, but it was his mother who took the lead, explaining that the family had had supper together at about six o'clock and that her son had then gone up to his room. At about ten o'clock she had gone up with a cup of coffee, and found him looking at his computer, but apparently having turned blue, and she had immediately dialled 999 for an ambulance. There was no history of any serious illness, and he was not on any medications.

I then asked the patient if I could examine him. He didn't seem in any way distressed or breathless, but his whole skin was a rather strange and unnatural bright blue colour; blue, and certainly not the blue colour that patients have if they are cold or in shock or respiratory failure, and his lips and tongue were a healthy pink. By this time, the ward sister to whom I had spoken a few minutes earlier had reappeared, and passed me, as requested, some gauze swabs which she had run under a warm tap. I rubbed one of the swabs on an area of blue skin on the thigh, and normal pink skin emerged. I looked at the swab, and it had turned blue.

The young man, without saying a word, rose from the bed, and walked off the ward, followed by his mother and father, who also remained silent, though the father still had an expression like thunder on his face. We never heard from them again, and what motivated the patient, we will never know. I can only speculate that it was a bizarre prank which got out of hand.

Attempts at simulating skin disease are not, in fact, that rare. Every dermatologist will see, from time to time, children brought to the hospital by an alarmed and distressed parent, who has discovered them covered in bright red patches of variable size and shape. The child is invariably perfectly well, usually has a cheerful smile, and appears to be enjoying the attention, and the parent is highly embarrassed, when the 'rash', created with paint or felt tip pen, is demonstrated to dissolve in water. More often than not, it turns out that the child is unhappy at school, and has found a clever way of getting a day off.[10]

Some patients presenting with a simulated or contrived skin disorder are more puzzling. Once a month there is a meeting in London of senior dermatologists from around the country where difficult or unusual diagnostic cases of patients with skin disorders are presented and discussed. I rarely miss a meeting. I vividly recall attending the meeting some years ago at which the dermatology team from a major teaching hospital in the north of England brought along a man who some months previously had turned a strange and somewhat unnatural shade of green. He had undergone every imaginable investigation which had failed to elucidate the cause.

The patient had cheerfully accompanied his doctors on the train down to London, which must have startled their fellow passengers.

He was a man was in his mid-twenties, appeared otherwise well, and seemed remarkably unperturbed by the doctors examining him. Eventually, one of my colleagues asked him about his occupation.

"Oh, I work in a shop," he replied.

---

10   There is an excellent account of the phenomenon in the autobiography of the champion jockey A.P. McCoy, who describes how he didn't enjoy school and from time to time painted himself with red spots and told his mother that he had chickenpox. It was only after a number of episodes that his mother discovered that children do not normally get repeated infections with chickenpox.

"What sort of shop?" my colleague persisted.

"A bookshop," he answered, mentioning the name of a well-known high street chain.

"And what do you do in the bookshop?"

"I work in the science fiction section," came the astonishing reply.

As far as I know, no one ever established what this man was doing to himself, unless of course, he had been abducted by aliens from outer space, emerging from one of his books. Perhaps he just had an overvivid imagination or a harmless practical joke had gotten a little out of hand.

There is one quite remarkable and difficult category of self-inflicted skin disease which is altogether more challenging for the dermatologists to whom it presents, and this is termed *dermatitis artefacta*. These patients, for reasons unknown, contrive to produce lesions on the skin, and then present to doctors claiming complete ignorance as to their cause. One must presume that there is a psychological background, or in some cases an attempt to evoke sympathy or obtain compensation, but these patients resolutely deny any knowledge of how their skin problem arose. If challenged, they tend either to walk out, loudly announcing that they are going to find 'a proper doctor', or attempt to prove you wrong by reattending the clinic with even more dramatic lesions.

The diagnosis is often rather obvious, with marks on the skin having a geometrical pattern or linear distribution which simply would not occur in any 'naturally occurring' disease. Lesions may be produced in various ways, such as by the application of alkalis or acids to the skin, or by injecting noxious agents. The patient invariably expresses complete bafflement.

I recall one middle-aged lady from early in my career who presented with ulcerated lesions arranged in odd geometrical patterns on the left arm and right leg. We admitted her to the ward for dressings, and the lesions healed, but identical marks then appeared on the right arm and left leg. When we bandaged both arms and both legs, identical marks appeared on the face. It eventually transpired that the injuries were caused by her injecting the skin with sour milk.

Dr Alan Lyell (1917-2007) was a distinguished Scottish dermatologist who worked at the Glasgow Royal Infirmary. He wrote some classic papers on dermatitis artefacta, which I would recommend to anyone who is interested in the topic. One of his papers[11] begins with these words, which will ring true to any dermatologist who has dealt with such patients. *'The idea that our patients are doing everything in their power*

11   A. Lyell, Dermatitis Artefacta and Self-Inflicted Disease. Scottish Medical Journal 1972, volume 17, 187. Dr Lyell's greatest contribution to medicine was to identify a condition called Staphylococcal Scalded Skin Syndrome. This is almost the exact opposite of Dermatitis Artefacta, in which children present with lesions which look like burns or scalds, but which in fact are caused by a strain of Staphylococcus which produces a toxin which destroys the outer layers of the skin. Until the condition became well recognised, there had been cases in which the parents had been falsely accused of child neglect or of non-accidental injury.

to help us make them better is so deeply ingrained in us that it comes as something of a shock to discover that some are pitting their wits against ours in a campaign of lies and deceit.'

The saddest case of dermatitis artefacta that I have encountered in my career was a young man with an ulcer on his foot which persistently failed to heal. He was seen by several dermatologists and extensive investigations were undertaken which excluded any 'naturally occurring' skin disease. The ulceration continued to progress despite the assiduous efforts of our nursing staff. The mystery was resolved when one of the nurses, when changing his dressings, found a number of sharp shards of broken plastic which had clearly been recently inserted into the wound.

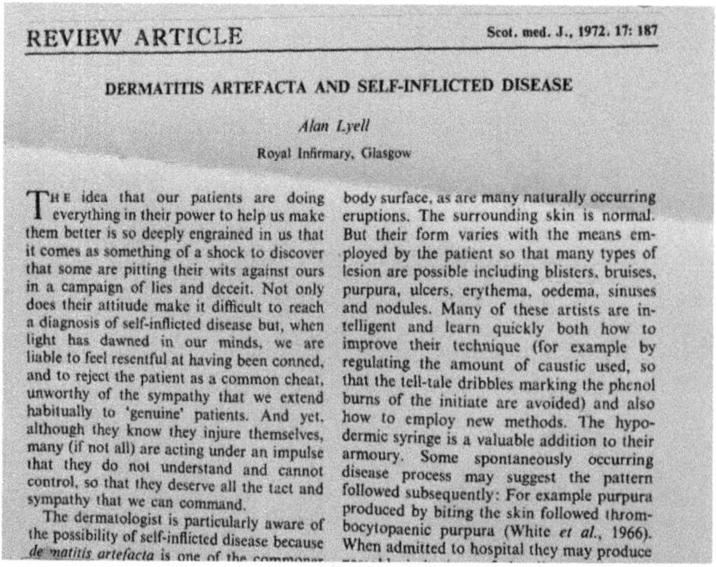

REVIEW ARTICLE

Scot. med. J., 1972. 17: 187

DERMATITIS ARTEFACTA AND SELF-INFLICTED DISEASE

Alan Lyell

Royal Infirmary, Glasgow

THE idea that our patients are doing everything in their power to help us make them better is so deeply engrained in us that it comes as something of a shock to discover that some are pitting their wits against ours in a campaign of lies and deceit. Not only does their attitude make it difficult to reach a diagnosis of self-inflicted disease but, when light has dawned in our minds, we are liable to feel resentful at having been conned, and to reject the patient as a common cheat, unworthy of the sympathy that we extend habitually to 'genuine' patients. And yet, although they know they injure themselves, many (if not all) are acting under an impulse that they do not understand and cannot control, so that they deserve all the tact and sympathy that we can command.

The dermatologist is particularly aware of the possibility of self-inflicted disease because dermatitis artefacta is one of the commonest body surface, as are many naturally occurring eruptions. The surrounding skin is normal. But their form varies with the means employed by the patient so that many types of lesion are possible including blisters, bruises, purpura, ulcers, erythema, oedema, sinuses and nodules. Many of these artists are intelligent and learn quickly both how to improve their technique (for example by regulating the amount of caustic used, so that the tell-tale dribbles marking the phenol burns of the initiate are avoided) and also how to employ new methods. The hypodermic syringe is a valuable addition to their armoury. Some spontaneously occurring disease process may suggest the pattern followed subsequently: For example purpura produced by biting the skin followed thrombocytopaenic purpura (White *et al.*, 1966). When admitted to hospital they may produce

Figure 4: Lyell's 1972 paper is well worth reading. Little more is known on the subject fifty years on.

The patient immediately discharged himself, but he subsequently found himself under the care of a surgeon who agreed, despite my words of caution, to the patient's request to perform an amputation. I was then called to the surgical ward as a matter of urgency a few days later as he had developed some ulcerated lesions on his head. Careful examination revealed more shards of plastic. I explained as sympathetically as I could, that this was a bad idea, as we wouldn't be able to amputate his head. He discharged himself a few days later, and we were never able to find out about his subsequent progress, nor what had motivated him.

It is easy to simply regard these patients as time wasters, but one has to reflect on the fact that they must all, in some way or another, be deeply troubled. The frustrating thing is that they present in a way that makes it very difficult to help them. To quote, once again, Dr Lyell, *'Not only does their attitude make it difficult to reach a diagnosis of self-inflicted disease but, when light has dawned in our minds, we are liable to feel resentful at having been conned, and to reject the patient as a common cheat, unworthy of the sympathy that we extend habitually to 'genuine' patients. And yet, although they know that they injure themselves, many (if not all) are acting under an impulse that they do not understand and cannot control so that they deserve all the tact and sympathy that we command.'*

CHAPTER FOUR

THE HUMAN GUINEA PIGS

The Covid pandemic has had a major effect on dermatology. Coronavirus infection can cause skin problems, some of a type that we have not previously encountered, and it can aggravate common skin disorders such as eczema and psoriasis. Additionally, of course, almost everyone has been under a lot of stress, and stress can certainly have an impact on the skin[12]. On top of all that, patients have found it difficult to get access to their GP, and it is impossible to make diagnoses of skin problems over the telephone. I mention all this to explain why I have been busier in my private practice than I have ever been.

A few months ago, I was in my clinic and had finally reached my last patient, an eleven-year-old girl. Her mother explained that her daughter had had an itchy rash for several months. All sorts of treatments had been tried, blood tests performed, and nothing seemed to have helped. The itching kept the child awake at night so that she was too exhausted to stay alert at school, and the whole situation was clearly getting the family down. I explained to the girl that I would like to look at her skin so that I could see if I could work out what the problem

---

12   See Chapter One, 'Going Like a Bomb'.

was. I asked if she would go with my nurse, undress down to her pants and vest and lie down on the examination couch.

She turned to her mother and said, "I'm not getting undressed," and despite her mother's pleading, she still refused. It had been a very long and challenging day. I was tired and my natural inclination was just to say 'goodbye', but I gently persisted, and eventually, with a certain amount of bad grace, the child acquiesced.

I always examine the skin in a systematic fashion, starting with the hands, including the fingernails, then the arms, and then the whole of the body, starting at the top of the head and working downwards. The poor girl's skin was covered in scabs and scratch marks, where she had been itching. No wonder she was feeling miserable. It was only when I reached the soles of her feet that the diagnosis became obvious. There were the little serpiginous, slightly scaly burrows, each with a tiny greyish dot at its front, that are diagnostic of scabies.

I turned to the mother. "I know what the answer is, and it's something that we can sort out, but may I ask a question? Has anyone actually looked at the skin like I have just done?"

The girl's mother explained that there had been numerous telephone 'consultations', sometimes with a doctor, more often with the practice nurse, but no, no one had actually looked at her skin. Dermatology isn't always easy, but if you don't examine the patient, it is even more difficult.

Scabies is an infection of the skin caused by a tiny, eight-legged mite, *Sarcoptes scabeii*. The mite burrows under the skin, where it lays its eggs and leaves behind its droppings. At night it emerges from its burrow and wanders over the skin until it finds another congenial point to burrow into the skin. In the initial phase, the condition is completely asymptomatic, but after about two weeks, patients develop a sensitivity to the mite's debris, and this causes furious and unremitting itching, worse at night. In turn, the itching provokes scratching, and the scratching causes breaks in the skin which are susceptible to secondary bacterial infection.

Occasionally patients, or their parents, are reluctant to accept the diagnosis. The simplest and most reliable way to convince them is to gently remove a mite from its burrow with a needle, place it on a microscope slide, and show the patient. The mite usually obliges by waving its antennae from the other end of the microscope. On one memorable occasion, I carefully removed a mite, placed it onto a slide, and put the slide on the microscope. I rushed off to find a couple of medical students who were in the department for the afternoon, but by the time I returned, the mite had wandered off in search of a more agreeable location. I spent a few weeks worrying that our cleaning lady might catch scabies, but fortunately, she didn't.

Scabies has been recognised for hundreds of years, and for a very long time it was attributed, erroneously, to poor personal hygiene. One curious, and still unexplained feature of scabies is that its prevalence waxes and wanes. As a dermatologist, you may not see a case for three or four years and then, all of a sudden, you are seeing several cases every day.

At the beginning of the Second World War, scabies was going through one of its upward phases in Britain and was particularly prevalent in the Armed Forces. By the time of the evacuation of Dunkirk in 1940, about five percent of British soldiers were said to be affected, and more soldiers were unfit for service because of scabies than because of war wounds. A man who is infected with scabies, and who can't sleep at night because of itching, is unlikely to be an efficient soldier and would be an unpopular companion in a tent or a trench.

The military authorities blamed poor hygiene, the conventional view at the time. Army laundry services were run night and day, boiling towels, bedding and uniforms, but scabies infections continued unabated. Fortunately, they sought the assistance of a remarkable man, Kenneth Mellanby, an insect biologist, who conducted an extraordinary series of human experiments on a group of Conscientious Objectors[13] who had volunteered to assist him.

Mellanby's intrepid group of 'human guinea pigs'[14] were housed in a large ramshackle property in Sheffield. They had a spacious garden in which they grew much of their own food and were kept isolated from the general population.

---

13   Conscientious Objectors were people who refused, on moral grounds, to join the Armed Services. They were required to do other work, often of a menial nature, such as working as cleaners or porters in hospitals. Some joined the services in 'non-combat' roles, including the bomb disposal services.
14   'Human Guinea Pigs' is the title of the book written by Mellanby in 1945, recounting the story.

First of all, Mellanby artificially transmitted scabies to some of the group. He was able to show that, without treatment, scabies continued whether the subjects bathed and changed clothes every day or were denied a bath or fresh clothes and bedding for up to two months.

Then he demonstrated that scabies was not caught by people using the same towels, clothing or bedding, as subjects with scabies. He even got his guinea pigs to wear the un-laundered underclothes and pyjamas that had been worn the day before by subjects with scabies, or to use the same bedding or sleeping bags.

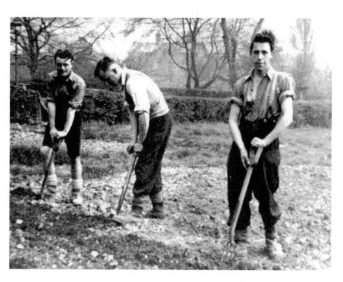

Figure 5: Three of Mellanby's 'guinea pigs', at the house in Sheffield.

Finally, in the crucial experiment, he showed that scabies was transmitted from person to person if they slept together in the same bed. He was rather coy in his account as to whether the guinea pigs were required to have sexual intercourse.

Crucially he also showed that treating the skin with a solution of benzyl benzoate[15] rendered patients 'non-infectious' within thirty minutes, although the itching may persist for a further couple of weeks.

Mellanby's conclusion, which remains our standard view, was that in adults, scabies is generally sexually transmitted; in young children, we believe that child-to-child transmission may occur innocently in the rough and tumble of play. He published his findings in the British Medical Journal (Figure 3) and subsequently in a book, aptly titled 'Scabies', which thanks to wartime restrictions was produced on very flimsy paper and in tiny font size. A facsimile edition in the original format was produced in 1972 and is compulsory reading for every dermatologist in training.

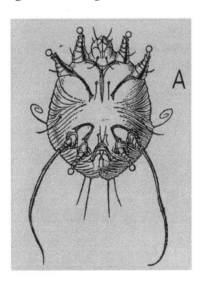

Figure 6: Adult scabies mite, from Mellanby's 1943 book, Scabies.

---

15   Less unpleasant agents are used nowadays in the UK, but benzyl benzoate is still widely used in the third world.

By present-day standards, Mellanby's experiments sound gruesome, and I doubt that they would get approval from a hospital medical ethics committee, but after the War, many of the 'guinea pigs' were interviewed and spoke highly of Mellanby and were grateful for the opportunity to have been able to contribute usefully to the war effort as non-combatants.

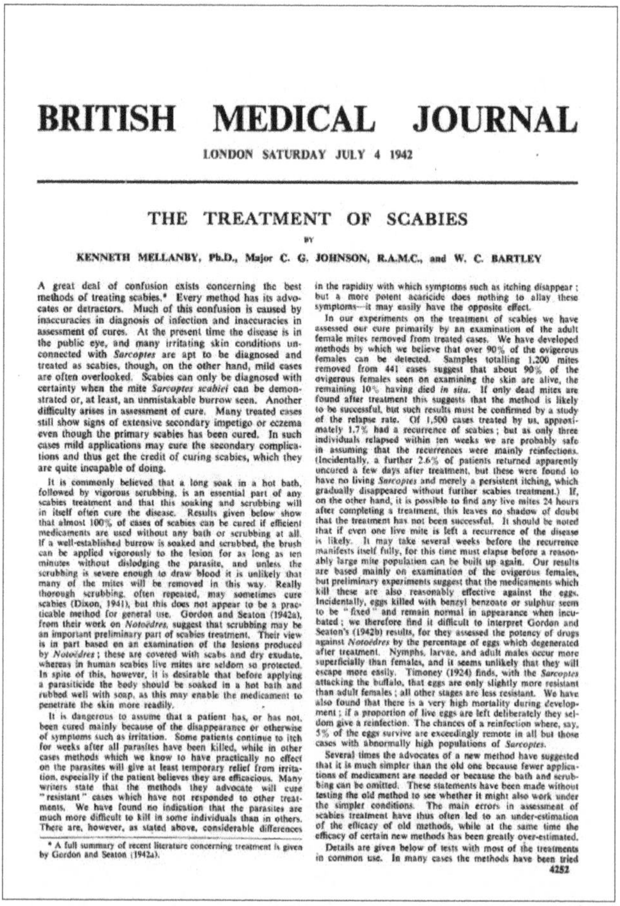

BRITISH MEDICAL JOURNAL

LONDON SATURDAY JULY 4 1942

THE TREATMENT OF SCABIES

BY

KENNETH MELLANBY, Ph.D., Major C. G. JOHNSON, R.A.M.C., and W. C. BARTLEY

A great deal of confusion exists concerning the best methods of treating scabies.* Every method has its advocates or detractors. Much of this confusion is caused by inaccuracies in diagnosis of infection and inaccuracies in assessment of cures. At the present time the disease is in the public eye, and many irritating skin conditions unconnected with *Sarcoptes* are apt to be diagnosed and treated as scabies, though, on the other hand, mild cases are often overlooked. Scabies can only be diagnosed with certainty when the mite *Sarcoptes scabiei* can be demonstrated or, at least, an unmistakable burrow seen. Another difficulty arises in assessment of cure. Many treated cases still show signs of extensive secondary impetigo or eczema even though the primary scabies has been cured. In such cases mild applications may cure the secondary complications and thus get the credit of curing scabies, which they are quite incapable of doing.

It is commonly believed that a long soak in a hot bath, followed by vigorous scrubbing, is an essential part of any scabies treatment and that this soaking and scrubbing will in itself often cure the disease. Results given below show that almost 100% of cases of scabies can be cured if efficient medicaments are used without any bath or scrubbing at all. If a well-established burrow is soaked and scrubbed, the brush can be applied vigorously to the lesion for as long as ten minutes without dislodging the parasite, and unless the scrubbing is severe enough to draw blood it is unlikely that many of the mites will be removed in this way. Really thorough scrubbing, often repeated, may sometimes cure scabies (Dixon, 1941), but this does not appear to be a practicable method for general use. Gordon and Seaton (1942a), from their work on *Notoëdres*, suggest that scrubbing may be an important preliminary part of scabies treatment. Their view is in part based on an examination of the lesions produced by *Notoëdres*; these are covered with scabs and dry exudate, whereas in human scabies live mites are seldom so protected. In spite of this, however, it is desirable that before applying a parasiticide the body should be soaked in a hot bath and rubbed well with soap, as this may enable the medicament to penetrate the skin more readily.

It is dangerous to assume that a patient has, or has not, been cured mainly because of the disappearance or otherwise of symptoms such as irritation. Some patients continue to itch for weeks after all parasites have been killed, while in other cases methods which we know to have practically no effect on the parasites will give at least temporary relief from irritation, especially if the patient believes they are efficacious. Many writers state that the methods they advocate will cure "resistant" cases which have not responded to other treatments. We have found no indication that the parasites are much more difficult to kill in some individuals than in others. There are, however, as stated above, considerable differences in the rapidity with which symptoms such as itching disappear; but a more potent acaricide does nothing to allay these symptoms—it may easily have the opposite effect.

In our experiments on the treatment of scabies we have assessed our cure primarily by an examination of the adult female mites removed from treated cases. We have developed methods by which we believe that over 90% of the ovigerous females can be detected. Samples totalling 1,200 mites removed from 441 cases suggest that about 90% of the ovigerous females seen on examining the skin are alive, the remaining 10% having died *in situ*. If only dead mites are found after treatment this suggests that the method is likely to be successful, but such results must be confirmed by a study of the relapse rate. Of 1,500 cases treated by us, approximately 1.7% had a recurrence of scabies; but as only three individuals relapsed within ten weeks we are probably safe in assuming that the recurrences were mainly reinfections. (Incidentally, a further 2.6% of patients returned apparently uncured a few days after treatment, but these were found to have no living *Sarcoptes* and merely a persistent itching, which gradually disappeared without further scabies treatment.) If, on the other hand, it is possible to find any live mites 24 hours after completing a treatment, this leaves no shadow of doubt that the treatment has not been successful. It should be noted that if even one live mite is left a recurrence of the disease is likely. It may take several weeks before the recurrence manifests itself fully, for this time must elapse before a reasonably large mite population can be built up again. Our results are based mainly on examination of the ovigerous females, but preliminary experiments suggest that the medicaments which kill these are also reasonably effective against the eggs. Incidentally, eggs killed with benzyl benzoate or sulphur seem to be "fixed" and remain normal in appearance when incubated; we therefore find it difficult to interpret Gordon and Seaton's (1942b) results, for they assessed the potency of drugs against *Notoëdres* by the percentage of eggs which degenerated after treatment. Nymphs, larvae, and adult males occur more superficially than females, and it seems unlikely that they will escape more easily. Timoney (1924) finds, with the *Sarcoptes* attacking the buffalo, that eggs are only slightly more resistant than adult females; all other stages are less resistant. We have also found that there is a very high mortality during development; if a proportion of live eggs are left deliberately they seldom give a reinfection. The chances of a reinfection where, say, 5% of the eggs survive are exceedingly remote in all but those cases with abnormally high populations of *Sarcoptes*.

Several times the advocates of a new method have suggested that it is much simpler than the old one because fewer applications of medicament are needed or because the bath and scrubbing can be omitted. These statements have been made without testing the old method to see whether it might also work under the simpler conditions. The main errors in assessment of scabies treatment have thus often led to an under-estimation of the efficacy of old methods, while at the same time the efficacy of certain new methods has been greatly over-estimated.

Details are given below of tests with most of the treatments in common use. In many cases the methods have been tried

* A full summary of recent literature concerning treatment is given by Gordon and Seaton (1942a).

4252

Figure 7: Mellanby's 1942 article in the British Medical Journal.

CHAPTER FIVE

JUMPING TO CONCLUSIONS

In dermatology, many conditions are of a chronic nature, or even lifelong, so if you stay in the same job as a consultant, you get to know patients quite well.

Mrs R[16] was an elderly farmer's wife. Her late husband, who had died a few years previously, had also been a long-standing patient. Farmers are interesting people to have as patients. They are instantly recognisable in the outpatient clinic by the 'two tone' skin on their faces, the lower half burnished to a reddy-orange glow by a lifetime of exposure to sun and wind, the upper half, protected by their hat, milky white and smooth.

They are also a stoical breed and don't make a fuss. They seem more comfortable than most with the idea of nature taking its course and of the natural cycle of life and death. Occasionally they can take this a bit too far. Another of my farmer patients, Mr F, a jolly man who always brightened up my clinic when he came to see me[17], managed to overturn his tractor. He crawled home, in great pain, and put himself to bed, refusing his

16   Throughout this book, I have changed people's names, and occasionally altered some details, in order to preserve patient confidentiality.
17   The first time I met him, he introduced himself with a memorable ditty: 'Bedfordshire born, Bedfordshire bred. Strong in the arm, Thick in the head.'

wife's suggestion that she call the doctor. He died in the night, having bled to death from a ruptured spleen and fractured pelvis. It was sad because his life could easily have been saved by prompt surgical intervention.

Mrs R was a delightful lady who had been a patient of mine over a number of years. She was always remarkably uncomplaining about her troublesome skin problem, but I had noticed that she had grown a little subdued since becoming a widow, and clearly missed her husband. I was seeing her for a routine follow-up consultation, and happened to notice her date of birth; it would be just a couple of weeks till her ninetieth birthday.

"I see that you have an important birthday coming up. Are you doing anything special?" I enquired.

"Oh yes," she replied, "I am going on a flight on an aeroplane. I've never been on one."

"Goodness, how lovely," I said. "Where are you going?"

"I am going to Zurich," she answered with a warm smile. "I am really looking forward to it."

"Well, I hope that you have a nice trip," I said and returned to the matter at hand, her skin problem. At the end of the consultation, I said that we would send her a follow-up appointment for three months' time, and off she went.

After she had gone, I began to think about our conversation. I could imagine someone wanting to fly in an aeroplane if they had never done so, but Zurich seemed a slightly strange choice. I have been there a few times, and it has always struck me as a rather sombre, Calvinistic sort of place. If you had never flown or been abroad, wouldn't you choose Paris, or Rome or Amsterdam, or indeed anywhere that would put a smile on your face?

Somehow, the matter preyed on my mind. Zurich had been in the news rather a lot in the preceding months. That in itself is somewhat unusual because in general, the good citizens of Zurich are very dependent for their wealth on private banking, an industry which relies on secrecy and discretion, and they try very hard to keep out of the news. What had brought Zurich to the front page of our newspapers was the establishment in 1998 of a clinic in the city called Dignitas, which was offering 'assisted suicide', something which is entirely legal in Switzerland.

In the United Kingdom, suicide was illegal until parliament passed 'The Suicide Act' in 1961. Until that time, a person attempting suicide could, if they failed, be charged with a criminal offence. Even after 1961, it remained against the law to assist another person to kill themselves. After the establishment of the Dignitas clinic, there had been a number of high-profile cases of individuals who had travelled from the UK with the purpose of being allowed to be assisted to die. There had also been a number of people in the UK suffering from incurable illness who had applied to the courts seeking to ensure that if their condition deteriorated to a degree that their life was, in their view, not worth living, their relatives or carers would not be prosecuted for assisting them to die. The British courts have never acceded to such requests, but these cases had propelled the subject of assisted suicide and the Dignitas clinic in Zurich into the limelight.[18]

Over the course of the next few days, my conversation with Mrs R kept coming back to me, and for some inexplicable reason, I managed to convince myself, without the slightest evidence, that Mrs R was going to Zurich to visit Dignitas. Why else would an elderly lady go to Zurich and she had used the word 'flight' in the singular, implying a one-way trip.

Three months later, I was sitting in my outpatient clinic, and looking through the list of patients. I noticed Mrs R's name, and said to my nurse, 'I don't think that the ten-thirty patient will be coming; perhaps I could have a cup of coffee.'

But I never got my coffee break because at ten-thirty, in came Mrs R, with her usual cheerful smile.

I asked her how her flight had been. "Oh, it was wonderful, Dr Monk. I can't wait to fly again."

"May I ask you a question? What made you choose Zurich as a destination?"

"Well," she explained, "my granddaughter lives there, and I wanted to see her."

---

18 'Assisted suicide' is an important subject on which people have strong views. I hope that no one is offended by this story, which I merely recount as it happened.

Somehow, I managed to hide my embarrassment, and we discussed her skin condition. In fact, it was going through a good phase, and we agreed that she would come again if she needed to but wouldn't book a fixed follow-up appointment.

It was about two years later that Mrs R's son, a jovial man of about sixty, who had taken over the running of the family farm, came to see me as a patient. We discussed his problem and I examined him and advised on the diagnosis. Then I enquired after his mother. I was delighted to hear that she was doing well, albeit getting a little frail. "She sends you her regards. She misses coming to see you".

"Don't tell your mother this," I said to him, "but I am going to tell you a story," and proceeded to recount the tale of how I had added two and two and made five.

He was a large man, as many farmers are, well over six feet tall and at least twenty stones, and was perched on the rather small chair that was provided for patients in the outpatient clinic. By the time I reached the end of my account, he was so convulsed with laughter that I thought that the chair was going to give way under him. When he had recovered his composure, he got up and said "Mother will love that story, I am going straight home to tell her."

A couple of years later, I received a lovely letter from the family, telling me that Mrs R had passed away, and thanking me for my care for her over the years. I seemed to have gotten away with it.

CHAPTER SIX

A THORNY PROBLEM

One of the most extraordinary achievements of medicine in the last hundred years is that thanks to immunisation, many previously fatal infectious diseases have been virtually eradicated, certainly in the Western world. Diphtheria, poliomyelitis and smallpox, all previously dreaded killers, are now rarely if ever, seen. Congenital rubella, a condition associated with severe lifelong handicap, and caused by German measles infection during pregnancy, has also, thankfully, all but vanished.

Tetanus is another condition which was once widespread and commonly fatal. It is caused by a bacterium, *Clostridium tetani*. The spores of this organism are widely distributed in soil, especially if it is wet, and in particular where there has been a lot of horse or cattle manure. It can be accidentally inoculated through the skin by an injury such as a garden fork or a thorn or by shrapnel from an explosion; this explains the high levels of tetanus in the First World War, especially in northern France, where so many battles took place on agricultural land[19]. In Britain, the highest incidence used to be in the fertile farmlands of East Anglia. Once inoculated, if

---

19   Tetanus was also very common in the American Civil War for similar reasons.

there is tissue damage reducing the levels of oxygen, the spores turn into the active bacteria which produce a nerve poison with similar characteristics to strychnine. In bygone days, it was called 'lockjaw' because one of the presenting features is a violent spasm of the jaw muscles, making it impossible for the patient to open their mouth. It is now so uncommon that few doctors have ever seen a case, but I still recall the patient who I admitted as a very young doctor.

In 1976, I was a house physician in medicine at Addenbrooke's Hospital, Cambridge, the most junior rank in the medical hierarchy. Mrs D was sixty and had been transferred to our ward from a small cottage hospital in the Fens, where she had been admitted for a routine minor operation.

Mrs D had worked at the hospital cooking and serving the lunches in the doctors' dining room for some thirty years. Because he knew her well, the anaesthetist who was due to assist with the operation decided to visit her on the ward before she went down to the operating theatre. After some initial chit-chat, he explained that he was going to give her a brief check-over. "Open your mouth, please," he directed.

Her mouth opened a fraction, and she began to explain that she couldn't open it any wider. The problem, it transpired, had started a couple of days earlier, and she was beginning to experience painful and violent muscle spasms in other parts of the body. There was a history of her having pricked her finger a few days earlier while pruning the roses in her garden. It later emerged that her husband, a keen gardener, had recently applied a generous quantity of horse manure to the rose beds.

The diagnosis of tetanus is essentially a clinical one, rather than one based on laboratory tests, but in Mrs D's case, I was able to carefully remove a rose thorn from her finger and rushed down to the laboratory with it. *Clostridium tetani* can only be grown in the lab in anaerobic[20] conditions, and fortunately, I had got my specimen to the microbiologists quickly enough for them to prove that this was indeed the culprit.

Although immunisation with Tetanus toxoid is highly effective in preventing tetanus, it has no effect in an established case. Mrs D's muscle spasms grew more violent and one of them threw her out of bed, breaking her arm as she landed on the floor. She needed artificial ventilation in the Intensive Care Unit, penicillin to kill off the causative bacteria, and administration of anti-tetanus serum, which binds to the tetanus toxin and neutralises it. She had a prolonged admission but went home and back to work cooking the doctors' lunches. A few weeks later she sent me a letter of thanks.

Nowadays, as a result of childhood immunisation, tetanus has been all but eliminated in the UK. We were never quite able to work out why Mrs D developed it after her rose thorn episode, but we suspect that she was too old to have been immunised as a child, and somehow missed out on subsequent immunisation. Sadly, tetanus remains common in many poor and underdeveloped parts of the world, especially in some parts of Africa and Asia where it is traditional for babies

---

20   Oxygen deprived

to have their umbilical stumps dressed with cow dung. This type of neonatal tetanus is invariably fatal, and it is terrible to think of babies dying needlessly from an entirely preventable condition.

CHAPTER SEVEN

IT'S A JUNGLE OUT THERE

Much of my training in dermatology was undertaken at King's College Hospital in South East London. It was a brilliant place to learn the subject, with a huge clinical workload and outstanding mentors to guide me. The surrounding catchment area has in recent years gone quite 'upmarket', but when I was there, much of it was a somewhat neglected inner-city part of London. Peckham, made famous by the TV series *Only Fools and Horses*, was just down the road. Elephant and Castle and The Old Kent Road, with their high-rise blocks, and doubtful pubs, (including the Thomas a Becket, and its famous boxing gym), were on our doorstep. It was home territory for one of London's most notorious crime gangs; the daughter of one of its leading lights was our outpatient receptionist and ensured that patients were always on their best behaviour.

To use an old expression, one could reasonably say that 'it was a jungle out there', but one of my most memorable patients from those days had literally emerged straight from the jungle.

Mr P was a twenty-five-year-old man who had just returned from several months working in the Amazon jungle, where he had been employed on a mapping expedition on the

Urubamba River[21], a remote and rarely visited area. He had previously been in the army, where he had trained as a surveying technician. Needless to say, it had been very hot and humid, and access to bathing facilities was limited. He had been subjected to innumerable insect bites and scratches in the course of his stay, but he had a number of places on the skin where deep ulcers had formed and which, even after his return to a more temperate climate, had continued to enlarge.

On examination, he appeared to be generally fit and well, but he had a number of deep ulcerated lesions on his skin, between two and three centimetres in diameter and with inflamed margins. One was on his forehead, one on his thigh and the others were on his trunk. The obvious thing to consider was whether Mr P had acquired some exotic skin disorder on his travels.

One important diagnosis at the top of our list of differential diagnoses was a condition caused by a protozoan and transmitted by sandfly bites called cutaneous leishmaniasis. In the early 1980s, the British Army had established a jungle warfare training centre in Belize[22], in Central America, and a steady stream of soldiers had been repatriated to the UK with the disorder, typically presenting as large non-healing ulcers of the skin[23]. Most of these cases had been managed by army dermatologists, but a number had been presented at clinical

---

21   I recommend that every doctor, and especially every dermatologist, should keep an atlas in their clinic.
22   Formerly British Honduras.
23   From 1981 to 1993, 306 British soldiers acquired leishmaniasis in Belize (Hepburn NC et al, British Journal of Dermatology (1993) volume 125, pages 63-68)

dermatology meetings or photographs shown in lectures, so although neither I nor my consultant had previously diagnosed a case, we were familiar with the appearance.

A skin biopsy was taken, and under the microscope, the pathologist, suitably forewarned of the possible diagnosis, was able to identify the characteristic intracellular inclusions, known as Leishman-Donovan bodies, diagnostic of leishmaniasis. Our clinical suspicion was confirmed.

Nowadays it would be possible to analyse the protozoan DNA by PCR[24] analysis, and this would have allowed immediate confirmation that this was one of the 'New World' leishmania species which untreated can spread to the nasal cavity and cause hideous destructive facial deformity. In the 1980s we had to make a clinical decision while awaiting rather more cumbersome tests, and we admitted Mr P to the ward for treatment with a rather curious and old-fashioned remedy, intravenous antimony, in the form of sodium stibogluconate[25].

---

24   PCR (polymerase chain reaction) is a technique used to amplify tiny fragments of DNA to allow them to be analysed; it has been called 'molecular photocopying.'

25   Leishmaniasis does not respond to conventional antibiotics.

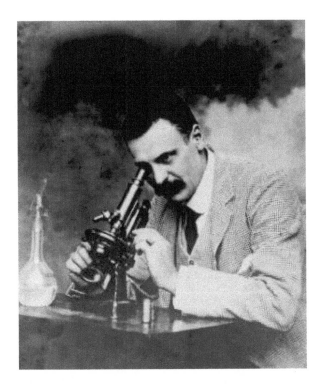

Figure 8: Major Charles Donovan of the Indian Medical Service,
who first identified the causative organism of leishmaniasis,
(by permission of the Wellcome Collection).

This uncommonly used drug requires monitoring of the patient for cardiac irregularities, but fortunately, he progressed well and the lesions began to heal. But there was another twist to the story. After about two weeks on the ward, Mr P pointed out a lump that had appeared on his thigh about 3cm in diameter. He had also noticed that there were three pinpoint openings on the surface, from which tiny air bubbles appeared at intervals. We watched incredulously, as none of us had seen anything like it.

I telephoned the duty doctor at the Hospital for Tropical Diseases at St Pancras, for further advice. He congratulated us on diagnosing leishmaniasis, but then said, "It's easily done, but you have made the first mistake in tropical medicine. Once you have made one diagnosis, keep looking for the next one," followed by the enigmatic advice, "Cover the holes with a layer of Vaseline and come back in the morning. The diagnosis will have emerged."

We felt as mystified as a visitor to the Delphic oracle, but we followed instructions, and next morning removed the dressing that we had placed over the lump, and there were three fat insect larvae, each about a centimetre in length, which had emerged overnight from their hiding place under the skin. Mr P had not only acquired leishmaniasis in the jungle but also a bizarre condition called myiasis. Cutaneous myiasis occurs in humans, or more commonly in cattle, when eggs of the botfly, *Dermatobia hominis,* (sometimes called 'the American warblefly')[26], laid under the skin of the host, develop into their larval form. When this stage is completed, they emerge and the skin lesion resolves. The remarkable thing is that the botfly actually lays its eggs on mosquitoes, and it is when the mosquitoes bite that the eggs penetrate the skin of the unfortunate victim.

The story of how leishmaniasis was discovered to be caused by a sandfly-borne protozoan is an interesting one.

---

26   Other flies are responsible for myiasis in Africa, but with a similar natural history.

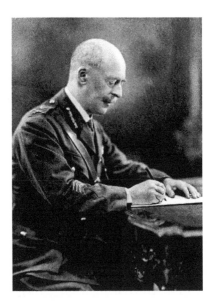

Figure 9: Sir William Leishman, after whom leishmaniasis is named (by permission of the Wellcome Collection).

In the late nineteenth century, Dum Dum in Western Bengal was a garrison town for the British Army in India. It was made notorious by the ordnance factory where 'dum dum' bullets, intended to expand on impact to cause maximum damage to the target, were first designed and manufactured[27]. Dum Dum was an unpopular posting, partly because it was a rather dismal town with a ghastly climate but also because many of the soldiers acquired an unpleasant and not infrequently fatal illness marked by fever, anaemia and massive enlargement of the spleen. The local Hindu name for the condition was *kala-azar*[28] but the British referred to it as 'Dum Dum fever'. Whatever anyone called it, the cause was entirely unknown.

---

27   They were made illegal in The Hague International Treaty of 1899.
28   Kala-azar means 'black skin'; in dark-skinned patients, deep pigmentation arises in longstanding cases.

In 1903, two army doctors, Dr Charles Donovan in India and Dr (later Sir) William Leishman in England, identified a parasite in tissue from patients with Dum Dum fever. Donovan demonstrated parasitic bodies in blood and spleen samples from sixteen patients, and Leishman found a parasite in post-mortem samples of the spleen from a soldier from Dum Dum who had died at a military hospital in Hampshire. In fact, Leishman incorrectly thought that what he was seeing were malaria parasites.

Donovan was keen to have the illness named 'donovaniasis' and Leishman was eager for it to be called 'leishmaniasis'[29]. Sir Ronald Ross, the man who had identified the malaria parasite[30] was asked to adjudicate. Leishman was the senior officer in the army, so Ross diplomatically suggested leishmaniasis, but the parasite was given the name *Leishmania donovani*, and the intracellular particles seen under the microscope are called 'Leishman Donovan bodies'.

Ross also established the natural history of leishmaniasis. It is essentially an infection of animals and is passed from one to another by sandfly bites. Man is only infected accidentally, and person-to-person transmission does not occur. Kala-azar, now known as visceral leishmaniasis, is a systemic disease in humans, but other Leishmania species cause ulceration of the skin at the site of the sandfly bites. Leishmaniasis is not

---

29   Donovan subsequently described a sexually transmitted disease caused by *Klebsiella granulomatis*. which was called 'Donovaniasis'.
30   Sir Ronald Ross (1857-1932) worked in the Indian Medical Service for twenty-five years and subsequently at the Liverpool School of Tropical Medicine. He established the cause of malaria in 1897, and received the Nobel Prize for Medicine in 1902.

uncommon in the Middle East, where it was formerly known by various names such as 'Oriental sore', 'Jericho boil' and 'Baghdad boil'. This form of the disease usually gets better on its own, although it tends to leave disfiguring scars at the site of the ulcers.

Other Leishmania species are found in Central and South America, the reservoir of infection usually being forest rodents. Effective treatment, as in Mr P's case, is essential to prevent catastrophic spread to the nasal and facial areas. Nearly forty years on, this is a case that I vividly remember.

As a footnote to anyone reading this who is a would-be traveller to exotic locations, leishmaniasis is still a condition to be avoided. Sandflies, which are the vectors of the infection, breed on stagnant water. They are tiny so they will easily penetrate a conventional mosquito net; sandfly-proof netting is of such fine calibre as to make sleeping almost impossible, so it is vital to cover the skin in a powerful insect repellent, re-applied at regular intervals. Sandflies are poor fliers, rarely venturing more than fifty metres from their breeding ground; they never venture above the height of a two-storey building, and can't fly well in more than the lightest breeze. So, sleep as high up as possible, and in as windy a spot as you can find. Local people have usually learned the places to avoid, so follow their advice.

CHAPTER EIGHT

ARE YOU SITTING COMFORTABLY?

Over time and with training, dermatologists acquire the skill of pattern recognition. Appreciating the subtleties of shape and colour and distribution is what enables us to distinguish the hundreds of different skin diseases that turn up in our clinics. But in the summer and autumn of 2006, patients started appearing with a strange but distinctive rash which had doctors all over the country scratching their heads, and patients scratching less dignified parts of their anatomy. It took many months of detective work before the puzzle was finally solved.

One afternoon, an excellent local GP called me. He had a patient in his surgery who, to use his words, was 'a horrible mess' and he had no idea of the diagnosis. I was in my outpatient clinic and I asked him to send the patient straight along.

Mr G was a man in his fifties, somewhat overweight but otherwise previously well. He had developed a rash which had gotten progressively worse over the course of a week. When I examined his skin the distribution of the rash was quite striking. There was a livid redness over the backs of his thighs, his buttocks, much of his back, across the back of his shoulders and the backs of his upper arms. In the affected areas, the skin was weeping and intensely painful, and he was clearly distressed. The rest of the skin was unaffected.

The appearance was very strange, and I really couldn't account for it at all. He hadn't used anything different in his bath or shower, hadn't been exposed to any chemicals at home, in the garden or at work, and hadn't done anything different in his life.

I don't like treating patients without a diagnosis, but Mr G was in quite a state, and I arranged for him to start a course of antibiotics and our nurses arranged daily application of a potent topical steroid. By the end of the week, he was no better, and the curious distribution of the rash was quite unchanged. No new areas of skin were involved.

He was in such discomfort that I admitted him to hospital. An extensive range of investigations were all negative and a skin biopsy showed changes of severe dermatitis but with no clue as to the cause. His condition cleared over the course of a few days and he went home, but three days later he phoned me, saying that the problem was worse than ever and that his wife was now affected, not quite as badly, but in exactly the same places on her skin.

I asked him to come back to see me, and as he walked into the room, he greeted me with the words "It's that bloody sofa. I told her there was nothing wrong with the old one."

He explained that at his wife's request they had bought a new green leather sofa from a well-known retailer just a few days before the problem started. The distribution of the rash, over the back of the thighs, buttocks, central back, shoulders and backs of the arms, fitted exactly where it had come into contact with the skin. The improvement when he came into hospital and the relapse when he went home was further evidence, and it seemed that his wife spent much less time watching television than he did, which might explain why she had less of a problem.

But I still didn't have a proper explanation as to why they had reacted in this way. Plenty of people have leather sofas, but I had never encountered anything like this. Occasionally you encounter people who react to leather products if they develop sensitivity to chromates used to tan the leather, but the reaction would not come on so abruptly. It might be possible to react to furniture polish or cleaning products, but there was no relevant history.

I arranged to investigate Mr G further by patch testing, but before I had done so, he advised me that he had sold the sofa to, as he put it, 'some other mug'. He didn't want any more tests and just wanted to forget about the whole experience.

Shortly afterwards, I attended a national educational meeting for dermatologists, and in the lunch interval the sole topic of conversation was what people were calling 'sofa dermatitis'. Quite a number of consultants, from diverse parts of Britain, had seen cases almost identical to mine. Some had seen several, but others had seen none at all. Many had had cases severe enough to require admission, and in a few cases the pathology from biopsy specimens, when examined under the microscope, had shown such florid inflammation that the diagnosis of a lymphoma of the skin had been suggested.

The pattern of distribution of the rashes did, of course, fit with there being a connection with the sofas, the affected areas of the skin, the back of thighs, buttocks, back, back of shoulders and backs of the arms being the areas of skin that would be in direct contact. In a number of cases where patch testing had been undertaken looking for an allergic contact dermatitis, patients had reacted to samples of leather taken from the sofa, but there was still no explanation as to what was really going on.

Not long afterwards, articles, accompanied by suitably lurid photographs, appeared in a number of national newspapers, and this in turn seemed to generate more and more patients coming forward. Almost all gave the same story and had the same pattern of distribution of their rash. There were, however, a few cases involving babies and young children, who had rested on a sofa for a sleep and who had developed a similar pattern of rash on their faces. These were particularly distressing for those affected.

Nor did it take long before firms of solicitors, circling like vultures over a carcass, started taking notice, and adverts appeared in newspapers inviting affected individuals to contact them. The scale of the problem can be judged by the fact that I received a letter from a firm of solicitors asking if I could examine and prepare expert medical reports on five hundred people[31]. I politely declined, not least because neither I nor anyone else really understood what was actually going on.

It soon emerged that there was a similar outbreak of 'sofa dermatitis' in Finland, which seemed to have started some months before the UK cases had begun to emerge, and a few cases were diagnosed in the Republic of Ireland, though whether they had bought sofas in the United Kingdom was not clear. To add to the confusion, once the problem got into the public domain, there were a few people claiming to have become allergic to their sofas but who, it transpired, had entirely unrelated problems.

Resolving the problem took considerable detective work, most notably by a newly appointed consultant dermatologist at Whiston Hospital in Merseyside, Dr Sandra Winhoven. It was established that all reactions related to a single brand of sofas and reclining chairs manufactured by a company in China, LINKWISE, all at the same factory, and sold in the UK by just three retailers. Inside the sofas, sachets had been placed marked 'MOULDPROOF AGENT, DO NOT EAT'. The sachets had apparently been put in place by the manufacturer to inhibit mould affecting the leather whilst the furniture was in transit but they hadn't notified the retailers that it was intended that they should be removed before the product was put on sale.

---

31 Some two thousand people are thought to have brought legal claims; not all were successful, as one of the retailers involved went out of business before matters could be settled. It is likely that several thousand people were affected altogether.

The sachets contained a powder which was shown on analysis to be 97% composed of a chemical called dimethyl fumarate (DMF). DMF has a rather unusual chemical property in that it 'sublimates', that is to say, that when warmed it changes from solid directly to a gas without going through a liquid phase. Sublimation of DMF occurs just below body heat, and the warmth generated by sitting on the sofas was sufficient to produce a vapour which impregnated the leather.

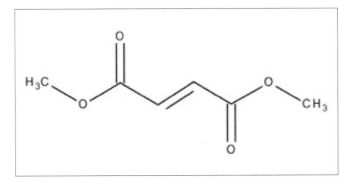

Figure 10: The culprit, Dimethyl fumarate.
A rather simple molecule to have caused such mayhem.

Testing of patients with 'sofa dermatitis' showed that their skin would react to concentrations of DMF as low as one part in a million, making DMF one of the most potent contact sensitisers ever discovered. Indeed at least one dermatologist managed to become sensitive to DMF just by performing patch testing on patients.

The story was featured on BBC television, with an episode of the consumer programme *Watchdog* being devoted to it. Once the problem was identified, the sofas were immediately withdrawn from sale, and those who had bought them were offered safer replacements or refunds. The problem vanished almost as soon as it had appeared, although the legal cases brought by victims rumbled on for several years. Then in 2011, there was an outbreak of 'shoe dermatitis' relating to leather shoes, again caused by DMF and again in a product made in China. Fortunately, by this time, dermatologists were alert to the issue and shortly afterwards, the EU banned the use of DMF in consumer products[32]. None of us has seen a case since.

---

32   Whatever one's opinion of Brexit, the EU did a great deal to help dermatologists and their patients, including introducing compulsory ingredient labelling of cosmetics and toiletries which assists patients with allergies, and the banning or restriction of a number of highly sensitising preservatives in personal care products. The EU also restricted the use of nickel in jewellery and other materials which come in contact with the skin, which has greatly reduced the prevalence of contact dermatitis to nickel.

CHAPTER NINE

PORRIDGE

One of my favourite television programmes is *Porridge*, starring that wonderful comic actor Ronnie Barker. Ronnie plays the part of an incorrigible criminal, Norman Stanley Fletcher, and the series is set in the fictional Slade Prison. The opening credits show a real prison, HMP Chelmsford, one of those typically grim and forbidding Victorian edifices. It is a building which bore a remarkable resemblance to Bedford Prison, a place which I passed on my way to work every day at Bedford Hospital[33].

Some months after I started work as a consultant, I was asked to see a patient who was a resident of Bedford Prison. He was a rather insalubrious character and had been remanded in custody for a serious violent offence. He arrived in the clinic handcuffed to two burly prison officers, but somehow his family had discovered details of his appointment, and when he arrived, his guards were surrounded by nine of his relatives who attempted, fairly vociferously, to persuade them to release him. A rather frightening fracas ensued, and he remained in custody, but thereafter whenever a dermatology appointment was required for a prisoner, I was summoned to go to the medical wing at the prison to see them.

---

33   By a curious coincidence, Ronnie Barker was born in Bedford.

I used to make a visit to the prison every few months. It wasn't too much of a chore and seeing a patient generated a modest fee payable by the Home Office, which at that time was responsible for prisons. In fact, whenever I arrived, the warders on the medical wing cheerfully announced that they had a second prisoner for me to see. Strangely, the second prisoner usually had little or nothing wrong with them, and eventually, I worked out that if I saw two patients, I was paid for a half day, a substantially larger fee than the one payable for seeing one patient. The second prisoner was usually happy, as it gave him a bit of variety from the usual dull routine, but it did make me wonder about the probity of the warders.

There was another strange ritual when you arrived. One of the favoured jobs for prisoners within any prison is to be an assistant in the medical wing. Their exalted status was demonstrated by the red armband that they wore on their blue prison uniforms. As soon as I arrived the 'red band', as they were known, would ask if I would like a cup of tea. It always seemed impolite to say 'no' and a large mug of some evil-looking liquid would appear. As soon as his back was turned, I poured it down the drain untasted, but shortly afterwards a second mug would appear, as it seemed that I must be thirsty as I had polished off the first one so quickly.

I suspect that *Porridge* has much to answer for, presenting the image of prison as being full of 'cheeky chappies' having a fun-filled break from the realities of life. In fact, it is grim, noisy and smelly, and the great majority of the prisoners who I met were poorly educated, frequently with dysfunctional family backgrounds and mental health, drug and alcohol problems.

The possibility of any meaningful 'rehabilitation' seemed remote.

Many of the cases which I saw were fairly mundane, but on one occasion I saw a thirty-year-old Polish man, who spoke virtually no English. I had no idea why he was in prison, and it was part of the etiquette that you didn't ask. He was smothered from head to toe with a very severe form of a disorder called psoriasis, which had come on quite abruptly a few weeks beforehand. Sometimes psoriasis can be aggravated or triggered by HIV infection. It was impossible to get any relevant medical history so I arranged for him to have an HIV test.

A few days later the hospital pathology lab contacted me to tell me that his blood result was positive. I phoned the prison to advise the medical wing of the result, only to be told that he had been discharged from prison and that there was no known address or mobile phone number. I felt awful for this poor chap who was unwell, didn't speak a word of English, and who needed medical treatment, but there was nothing I could do. Perhaps I am doing them an injustice, but I formed the distinct impression that the prison service couldn't have cared less; it was no longer their problem. Sadly, this wasn't the only occasion that I encountered this attitude, and I decided to decline any further kind invitations to see patients there.

A few years later, however, I did have another encounter with a prisoner. I undertake a certain amount of medicolegal work, and I received a letter from a firm of solicitors, asking if I could examine their client, a resident of Wormwood Scrubs prison in West London, who wished to sue the prison medical officer and the Ministry of Justice[34] for their alleged failure to provide adequate treatment for a severe condition affecting his skin and joints. A substantial fee was offered for my services.

I had never been instructed in a case anything like this and my curiosity was piqued. Before accepting instruction, I wanted to know a little more, and I entered the potential client's name into an internet search. Computers can be frustrating, but it is difficult to imagine how we managed before we could search for everything at a touch of a button. In this case, I hit the jackpot.

There were long articles in the *Daily Mail* and *Daily Telegraph* newspapers, revealing that the prisoner, Mr BB, was currently serving eight years at Her Majesty's pleasure (and taxpayers' expense) having been found guilty of a series of enormous, fraudulent medical claims, which had netted him a seven-figure sum.[35] He had sat in the dock throughout the trial in a wheelchair, claiming to be totally incapacitated. When the judge came to pass sentence, he told the prisoner that there was no medical reason for him to be in a wheelchair and that unless he stood up, he would give him an additional six months. To gasps of astonishment, he rose like Lazarus in the New Testament.

---

34   By this time the Home Office had passed responsibility for the prison service to the newly formed Ministry of Justice.

35   You can read about it here: https://www.telegraph.co.uk/news/uknews/crime/9511818/Wheelchair-faker-scammed-1.8-million-in-disabled-grants-to-fund-champagne-lifestyle.html

The *Daily Mail* also helpfully posted a photograph of Mr BB jumping from a diving board into the swimming pool of his villa in Spain which had been purchased with his ill-gotten gains. There was no sign of any restriction to his mobility, nor of the skin disorder that he had claimed caused such incapacity.

No doubt Mr BB was hoping to bring his new claim against the medical staff in prison, assisted by the fact that the doctors, following normal prison etiquette, had not asked him why he was in prison![36]

I sent a copy of the *Daily Mail* article to the solicitors and explained that I did not think it appropriate for me to act as an expert in the case. They never replied.

On one occasion I was asked to act as an expert for the defence in a criminal trial. The defendant had been arrested for allegedly playing with his private parts in a public place. He had told the policeman who arrested him that he had done no such thing but had experienced a severe itching feeling in his groin and had merely stopped to scratch the affected area. I was asked by his solicitor to examine him in order to establish whether there was any condition of the area in question which might cause him to be affected by a sudden and overwhelming need to scratch.

---

36   In my experience in Bedford, if you do ask you are told either that it was a case of mistaken identity or that they had a useless barrister. I never encountered anyone who felt inclined to repent their sins, though no doubt there are some.

He had been remanded in custody in Bedford Prison to await trial, and that is where I had to go to examine him. I was able to establish that he had an absent right testicle and an extensive surgical scar in the right groin area, relating to a surgical procedure some years before. When the case came to trial at Peterborough Crown Court, I gave my evidence and expressed the opinion that some scars do itch, and that the defendant's story was totally plausible. The prosecution case was probably not helped when the police surgeon, who had examined the defendant after his arrest, had failed to notice the absent testicle and the scarring.

I must admit that on the evidence that I heard, I was somewhat surprised when the jury returned with a unanimous guilty verdict. If having a sudden itchy feeling in an embarrassing part of your anatomy was going to get you arrested, then all of us would need to be a lot more careful.

It was only after the verdict had been announced that the prosecution was allowed to reveal that the defendant had a very long history of sexual offences, many involving children, and had only just been released on licence from a custodial sentence. The offence had taken place outside a bail hostel where he had been living following his release from prison following his conviction for a similar offence. He was sent back to prison for a further period. I felt rather foolish to have been taken in by his story. Clearly, the jury had had the wisdom or common sense to see through it all.

I have always found medicolegal work interesting, as no two cases are quite alike. The overwhelming majority of cases are civil rather than criminal and usually relate to claims of medical negligence. One of my very first cases related to a claim for a large sum of money brought by an aggrieved patient against a dermatologist in Hong Kong. The evidence was voluminous, the patient having sought second opinions from some twenty-three doctors in several countries. I had been engaged by the solicitors acting for the doctor; I still remember being amused by the name of the firm, Wong, Cohen and Patel, which I thought covered most possibilities.

I diligently ploughed through all the documentation, and couldn't convince myself that the doctor had done very much wrong, and was all set to fly out, all expenses paid, for ten days in the Hong Kong High Court, when at the last moment the patient abandoned their claim.

One of the things that has always amazed me about medicolegal cases is the length of time that they take[37]. Lawyers seem to have no sense of time, and of course, they charge by the hour, so the longer a case rumbles on, the more they earn. I am currently acting as an expert (for the defence) in a personal injury case which to date has lasted seven years, and the end appears nowhere in sight.

In another case, being pursued in the Northern Ireland High Court, I was approached by a firm of solicitors acting for the claimant, in 2017, asking whether I was able to assist them. The case seemed quite complex and rather sad, and I said that I was happy to help. I heard no more until 2021 when they

---

[37] Nothing seems to change. Charles Dickens addressed the same subject in 'Bleak House', published in 1853.

wrote again asking whether I was still available. I wrote back saying that I was, but that given the snail-like rate of progress to date, I couldn't guarantee that I would still be alive when the case came to court. I have heard no more.

At the time of writing, the problem of long waiting times in the NHS is much in the news. It must be a great source of anxiety to patients and their families and a source of frustration to doctors, but the waits seem short compared to those experienced by people trying to get justice through our legal system.

CHAPTER TEN

KEEP YOUR HAIR ON

I was a fairly newly appointed consultant, when Mr A, a pleasant, elderly man, walked into my outpatient clinic. The most striking thing about him was that he was wearing a somewhat bedraggled wig worn at a jaunty angle.

He had been referred by his GP with regard to an ulcerated lump that was growing on his scalp. When I examined him, having persuaded him, reluctantly, to remove the wig, his scalp was completely devoid of hair, and the whole area was scarred. On the top of his head was a lesion which was clearly a skin cancer of a serious type known as a squamous cell carcinoma. It had apparently been growing for some time.

Mr A explained to me that as a child he had had ringworm of the scalp, and had been subjected to a treatment which was then in vogue of X-ray irradiation of the affected area of the skin. This had cured him of his ringworm but had caused extensive scarring of the affected area with permanent baldness. He had worn a wig ever since, and never allowed anyone, not even his wife, to see him without it. No doubt it was his embarrassment that had inhibited him from seeking help sooner.

Scalp ringworm is a misnomer. It is not caused by a worm, but is a fungal infection, more correctly called 'tinea capitis'. It used to be very common, and almost exclusively seen in children, boys more frequently than girls. The fungus affects the scalp and the growing hairs, causing patches of inflammation and scaling in which the hairs break off, leaving bald areas of skin. The diagnosis can be made in the clinic by carefully removing a few affected hairs, and putting them on a microscope slide with a few drops of potassium hydroxide. The branching fungal hyphae are easily seen on low power magnification. The species of fungus can be determined by sending a sample to the laboratory, where over two or three weeks the fungal colony will grow, with different patterns of growth being seen with different organisms.[38] In most cases of scalp ringworm the affected hairs fluoresce when the scalp is examined under ultraviolet light, and this is a quick way of checking whole families, or classes of school pupils when there has been an outbreak of infection.

Scalp ringworm is usually caused by species of fungus which pass from person to person; when I was at school it was strictly forbidden ever to put on another pupil's school cap or to use anyone else's comb, for fear that we might pick up ringworm. For reasons which are poorly understood, if untreated, the condition resolves spontaneously at puberty, and it used to be very uncommon for adults to be affected.

---

38   This is important for distinguishing fungi which have been acquired from animals, such as pets or cows, from those which spread from person to person.

It was not long after the discovery of X-rays by Roentgen in 1895, that it was observed that irradiation of the skin would cause hair loss. Soon X-ray treatment was being offered to ladies as a new scientific means of treating excessive hair on the face and elsewhere, with people apparently oblivious to the potential risks.

The use of X-rays as a treatment for skin disorders was also enthusiastically pursued. Dr James Sequeira[39], a dermatologist at the London Hospital, was an early advocate. Scalp ringworm was a condition that was particularly prevalent in poor, overcrowded inner-city areas, and the London Hospital[40] in Whitechapel was in the heart of London's East End. Scalp ringworm was a notoriously difficult condition to treat, and Sequeira devised a regime of 'X-ray epilation' which was widely used from 1905 onwards.

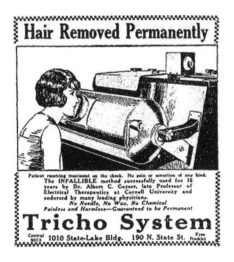

Figure 11: Early American advertisement for X-ray hair removal

---

39   1865-1946
40   Now the Royal London Hospital.

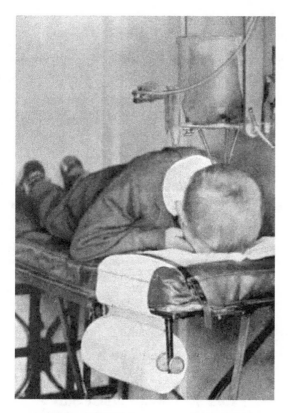

Figure 12: A child receiving X-ray epilation for ringworm at the
London Hospital. Sequeira's 'Diseases of the Skin' 1911.

The technique was to irradiate the scalp, and this was followed
a few weeks later by all the hair falling out and then, with time,
normal hair regrowing. Unfortunately, in those early days, it
was very difficult to calculate the dose of irradiation given, so
that in a proportion of cases, the scalp would be scarred, and
no hair would ever regrow. Sadly, there was a latent period
between the treatment and the hair fall, so sometimes, if the
doctor or the parents were impatient, a second treatment was
given, almost always with catastrophic results.

There were some doctors who remained apprehensive about the use of radiation as a treatment for children, and another method of epilation came into fashion using oral thallium acetate. Thallium is poisonous, with a very fine margin between therapeutic and fatal doses, so although it was an effective treatment, the outcome was not always satisfactory.[41]

It took much longer to recognise that not infrequently, and especially if there had been scarring, skin cancers could arise on the affected scalp often after an interval of many years, and indeed sometimes decades[42]. Nevertheless, the use of X-ray epilation for scalp ringworm was still being widely used until the late 1950s. For example, the Goldie Leigh Children's Hospital in South East London was treating several hundred children with scalp ringworm every year until 1959.

Mr A was one such victim, and his case was a challenging one. Squamous cell carcinoma of the scalp can normally be effectively treated by irradiation or by surgical removal. However, radiation is totally contraindicated in cancers which have been caused by X-rays, as in Mr A's case. Surgical removal is always very challenging in radiation-damaged skin because the wound often heals very poorly. Fortunately, I was able to invoke the assistance of my excellent plastic surgeon colleague, the late Mr Peter Mahaffey, who, with great skill, was able to remove the tumour and repair the defect. We even

---

41   Thallium is colourless, odourless and tasteless, so is an ideal poison, and has been used by a number of murderers, including Graham Young, a notorious mass murderer.

42   X-rays were also used as a treatment for acne, eczema, warts and a myriad of other conditions. Cases of skin cancer, often occurring many years later, were seen in all these conditions.

managed to persuade Mr A to abandon his wig. He purchased a rather natty trilby instead.

The end of X-ray epilation as a treatment for scalp ringworm came quite abruptly. Topical applications of ointments and creams had never been effective and fungi do not respond to conventional antibiotics. A drug called griseofulvin with antifungal properties had been discovered in 1939 but had initially found only limited application as a veterinary medication in cases of cattle ringworm. It was subsequently shown to be safe and effective in treating experimentally produced ringworm in guinea pigs, and on that basis, a study was undertaken in the dermatology department at King's College Hospital, London, in 1958 of its application in children with ringworm. It was found to be highly effective and remarkably free of adverse effects, and the results were published in *The Lancet*. The drug was subsequently licenced for use and marketed by ICI. The cost of the drug to the NHS for a full course of treatment was twenty-five shillings.[43]

The use of X-ray epilation with all its potential hazards was abandoned overnight. The Goldie Leigh Hospital closed in 1961. It is many years since I saw a patient with scarring and skin cancers on the scalp secondary to treatment of childhood ringworm.[44]

---

43 £1.25p. The cost of some new drugs nowadays can run into thousands of pounds.

44 The history of epilation at Goldie Leigh is recorded in the British Journal of Dermatology, 1967, Volume 79, 237-8.

There was a rapid decline in cases of scalp ringworm, and that should have really been the end of the story, but there is a curious postscript.

By the time I began training in dermatology, scalp ringworm had become quite uncommon. I was a senior registrar in dermatology at King's College Hospital in the 1980s . It was a busy department, serving a large inner-city catchment population, and yet in my final year there, 1987, we saw just one case. Then things changed, and over the next five years or so there was a dramatic increase in numbers. Nearly all the cases were in young boys, mostly between six and eight years old, and overwhelmingly they were from the local Afro-Caribbean population. Nearly all were infected with a species of fungus called *Trichophyton tonsurans* normally uncommon in the UK. Similar outbreaks were seen in Paris and other large cities with substantial black populations.

The dermatologists at King's noticed an additional factor, which was that all the boys had, shortly before they had become infected, been to the barber, and nearly all had had their hair shaved in a way that was fashionable at the time. A major public health campaign was undertaken, and barber shops were educated to disinfect their clippers and scissors between clients. The problem resolved as rapidly as it had arisen, and scalp ringworm is once more, quite uncommon.

By a curious coincidence, my own grandfather had, over a hundred years ago, run a barber shop in South East London. I am sure that he would have carefully cleaned his tools between each customer.

CHAPTER ELEVEN

WHAT'S MY LINE?

Many years ago, when I was growing up, television was in black and white and there were only two channels. There was a popular show called *What's My Line?* Members of the public were invited to mime an activity which they did at work, and a panel of 'celebrities' were invited to try to guess what they did for a living. It was great fun, and I was always astonished at the strange variety of occupations that people had.

Nowadays, such a programme simply wouldn't be possible because, as far as I can make out, most people have a job which involves them looking intently at a computer screen for hours on end, and you would have no idea what they were trying to do.

In many ways, of course, it is good that hardly anyone has to spend a working lifetime in some of the disagreeable jobs that many people used to do, but asking a patient about their work is often a most illuminating part of taking a medical history, and their past or present occupation can be the key to the diagnosis. I still remember, as a junior doctor working on a medical ward, examining a distinguished barrister who had been admitted with a puzzling respiratory problem. I noticed some curious black lines on his forearms and shoulders, and rather surprised him when I asked when he had worked down a coal mine.

"How did you know?" he asked me with a puzzled expression.

I explained that what I had observed was accidental tattooing with coal dust from minor friction or trauma, the marks sometimes being called 'collier's stripes' and almost universal in miners and ex-miners. From the end of the Second World War until 1948, because of labour shortages, conscripts could be sent to work in the mines, rather than serve in the military, and my patient explained that this was exactly what had happened to him[45]. Much to his and my surprise, his chest problem turned out to be a delayed consequence of his exposure to coal dust decades earlier.

In the years prior to automation, and before Britain closed much of its manufacturing base, and before health and safety was taken seriously, going to work was a hazardous business, and every industry seemed to have its own particular source of danger. Workers in the hat trade were liable to the effects of mercury poisoning, caused by the release of mercury vapour when the felt material was steamed. It resulted in the phrase

---

45   The scheme to conscript men (no women were sent) to work in the mines was devised by a Labour Minister, Ernest Bevin, and they came to be called 'Bevin Boys'. They were often badly treated by the miners, who resented their presence, and sometimes abused by the members of the public, who didn't understand why they weren't in uform. It was long a bone of contention among the Bevin Boys that they didn't receive any official recognition for their contribution to the war effort. In 2007, the Prime Minister, Tony Blair announced that they were to receive a veterans' badge.

'as mad as a hatter' and Lewis Carroll's 'Mad Hatter'.[46] Painters commonly developed 'wrist drop' through paralysis of the peripheral nerves as a result of long-term exposure to lead in paint[47].

During the Second World War, the Timex watch factory in Dundee was engaged in producing instruments for military aircraft. Young ladies were employed in the highly skilled work of applying luminous paint so that the dials could be read in the dark, and this paint contained radium. Although radium was known to emit radiation, the hazard was not appreciated. The women, called 'radium girls', used to lick the tip of their brushes to allow them to keep the point fine, and subsequently many of them developed mouth cancers or, in some cases, leukaemia.

In the Sherlock Holmes stories, the famous detective was often making observations about the tell-tale signs on people's skin, which sometimes allowed him to solve a puzzling case. In the second Holmes book, 'The Sign of Four'[48], Holmes tells Doctor Watson that he had written a short book on the subject of 'occupational marks on the hands.' Sherlock Holmes, of course, was a fictional character, but the author, Sir Arthur Conan Doyle, was a doctor who had graduated from Edinburgh University. One of the doctors who taught the medical students at that time was Dr Joseph Bell, a physician at the Edinburgh Royal Infirmary. Bell was a very distinguished

---

46   Alice's Adventures in Wonderland (1865) and Alice Through the Looking Glass (1871)
47   Lead was only finally banned in paint in the UK in 1992.
48   Published in 1890.

doctor and served as a personal physician to Queen Victoria when she was in Scotland. He was very popular with the students for his ability to make deductions about patients' occupations, personal habits and travels from meticulous observation of their skin. Conan Doyle freely acknowledged Bell as the inspiration for Holmes.

Sherlock Holmes' short book on 'occupational marks' may have been a work of fiction, but in 1955 Dr Donald Hunter, a physician at the London Hospital, produced an extraordinary book, over a thousand pages in length, called 'Diseases of Occupations'[49] which documented the remarkable range of conditions which arose through people's work. Over the years I have spent many happy hours reading it because it is a treasure trove of the extraordinary dangers that people have exposed themselves to in order to make a living.

One chapter which is of particular interest to a dermatologist is the description of the early use of X-rays. The London Hospital, where Hunter subsequently studied and then worked as a consultant, was one of the first hospitals to acquire an X-ray machine. The exposure time for a picture with the original primitive apparatus was lengthy, and hospital porters were employed to hold the films in place while the image was generated. There was little idea at the time of the potential hazards of radiation, and they all subsequently died from radiation-induced skin cancers on their hands.

---

49   It is still in print, in its tenth edition and called Hunter's Diseases of Occupations. It now has over a hundred contributing authors, but if you can find a copy of the 1955 version it is well worth browsing through it.

It must be said that even when Hunter's book was published in 1955, many of the conditions described, and indeed many of the occupations, had become rarities. I vividly remember how in 1975, when I took my final exams, seeing one of my fellow students in a state of distress after the clinical cases in surgery. He explained to me that he had been asked to examine a man with a lump on the centre of the chest, overlying the sternum. He was completely flummoxed; he had never seen anything like it and had no idea of the diagnosis. After an embarrassing silence, the examiner, clearly trying to be helpful said, "Perhaps it would be helpful if you asked the patient what his occupation is."

It turned out that the patient was a cobbler, but my poor friend was none the wiser. After a further period of silence, the examiner explained that the lump was a pre-sternal bursa, "caused by his holding his last."

"His last what?" replied my perplexed friend, unfamiliar with the word.

Mysteriously he passed the exam and subsequently became a distinguished consultant physician at a London teaching hospital. I spent several years doing dermatology clinics in Northampton, traditionally the shoe-making capital of England. I saw hundreds of people who had worked in the shoe trade, and never saw a patient with a cobbler's pre-sternal bursa.[50]

---

50   A bursa is a fluid-filled swelling arising over a bone at a point of friction, most commonly seen over the knee or elbow. A cobbler's last is a device used to fashion or repair shoes, and usually held against the chest.

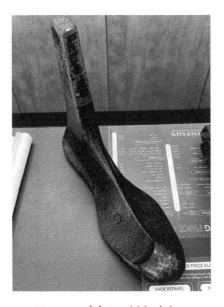

Figure 13 (a) A cobbler's last

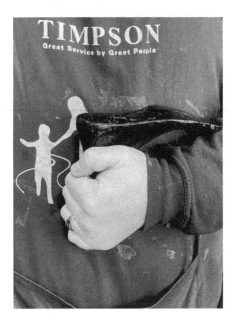

Figure 13 (b) A cobbler with his last, still in use in 2022. (Photograph taken with permission in Timpson's shoe-repairers, Bedford).

In the twenty-first century, dermatologists see few of the occupational marks with which Sherlock Holmes or Donald Hunter would have been so familiar. Nevertheless, carpet fitters can still always be recognised by the callosities over their knees and knuckles, and carpenters nearly always seem to be missing the tips of one or two fingers on their non-dominant hand. As mentioned in Chapter Five, farmers invariably have a remarkable two-tone colour to their faces.

Nevertheless, taking a good occupational history is vital. Where I practice is close to the headquarters of a number of the Formula One motor racing teams. The people who work there are invariably very pleasant and extremely bright, but until you get used to them can be challenging as patients. They are used to working to tiny fractions of a second, or to distances of a micron. In their work, these times or distances can be the difference between success and failure. If you suggest that they apply a cream once or twice a day for a few weeks, they look at you in puzzlement. It takes time to realise that they are much happier if you tell them to squeeze out one centimetre of cream and rub it in seven times in a clockwise direction at exactly 6 a.m. and 6 p.m. for twenty-one days.

A couple of years ago, I was just about to start my clinic when the phone rang. It was one of my regular patients who was the chief engineer for one of the top motor racing teams. He explained that he had an appointment with me that afternoon, but his car had broken down, and he wouldn't be able to get to see me. I reassured him and explained that I would be in the clinic all day and that he should just come along when he could.

He turned up a few hours later, and I asked him what had happened to his car. "Oh, I couldn't work out what the problem was, but a nice man from the AA got it going." I felt strangely reassured by my own lack of mechanical knowledge.

Patients' occupations can be relevant in all sorts of ways. A patient came into my clinic and sat down. He was in his forties and didn't look terribly well. He had had a temperature and a rash for about three weeks. I always try to work in a very methodical fashion and like to take the history before I start to examine the patient, but on this occasion, I was rather distracted from my usual routine, because from the moment he had sat down, I was sure, from the appearance of his face, that this was a case of secondary syphilis.[51]

Nevertheless, I carried on with my standard questions. I asked about his work, and he told me that he worked at a local airport.

"What do you do there?" I enquired, and he explained that he worked in security, checking what was in people's bags.

"How long have you done that?"

"Fourteen years." He replied.

"Have you ever found anything unusual in all the bags you

---

51   Secondary syphilis occurs several weeks or months after the initial infection and is highly infectious. The patient has a characteristic rash, patchy hair loss, fever, enlargement of lymph glands, and is generally unwell. If not recognised and treated, the patient will progress, often after some years, to tertiary syphilis, with brain and cardiac lesions.

have checked through?" I asked, for no particular reason. "No," he replied. I really couldn't think of anything worse than spending years doing a job like that.

I proceeded to examine him, and my initial impressions were confirmed. We don't see secondary syphilis every day, but if you have ever seen a case, you will never miss it. He had all the textbook features, including patchy hair loss[52], enlarged lymph nodes, a widespread rash, with the characteristic copper-coloured lesions on the palms and soles, and the so-called 'snail-track' ulcers on the tongue and mouth.

I explained the likely diagnosis and arranged blood tests and a skin biopsy, and saw him again a few days later with the results, which were positive.

"Had he any idea how he might have caught it?" I asked.

"Oh. It must have been something in one of those suitcases," he replied.

I am not sure that he was right; it certainly doesn't feature in 'Hunter's Diseases of Occupations.'

---

52   Always described in textbooks as 'moth-eaten.'

CHAPTER TWELVE

VLADIMIR PUTIN AND ME

As a dermatologist, I am well aware that we are often perceived, unfairly, of course, as largely dealing with trivialities. Sometimes one's medical colleagues think that we are not really proper doctors. And occasionally, when I have had one of those clinics when I have a succession of patients complaining that their eczema gets better when they use the treatment but comes back as soon as they stop, I am almost inclined to wonder whether I could be doing something more useful. But just once in a while, you find that you have made a rather bigger impact, literally, as you are about to read, than you could ever have imagined.

Some twenty-five years ago, I was contacted by the manager of a local factory, asking for my help. He explained that workers on a new production line were developing a severe and incapacitating rash. They were going off sick and were reluctant to come back, and it was causing the company real difficulties. I must say that he seemed less concerned about his employees than about the productivity of the factory.

I arranged to see about eight of them. They all gave the same story. In each case, the rash had started about six to eight weeks after they had started on a new production process. It improved if they were away from work, but came back as soon as they returned. The appearance of the skin was identical, with fierce eczema on the exposed areas of skin, the face, ears, neck down to the collar line, hands and wrists. Covered areas of skin were unaffected. The appearance was of an airborne contact dermatitis, and patch testing revealed a severe allergic reaction to an epoxy resin monomer.

Epoxy resins are best known for the 'two-phase' adhesives which are widely used in DIY and by model makers. They are also used to provide an impermeable surface, for example in boat building, furniture making, etc. The resin is mixed with a hardener which is a catalyst that makes the epoxy polymerise into an inert material. It is the 'uncured' epoxy monomer which commonly causes allergic reactions. Once the material has hardened, it is generally inert and harmless. Allergy to epoxy resins is not uncommon in people using the adhesives at home or at work and typically presents with eczema on the fingertips. Clearly, in the present case, something quite different was going on.

In those happy, far-off days I had more time than doctors do now, and I suggested that it would be helpful if I visited the factory to see what was going on. I still didn't know what the production process was all about. There was a short delay, which I subsequently discovered was while the factory obtained clearance from the Ministry of Defence for me to be allowed to visit.

When I finally did get to the factory, the manager explained to me that they were making a new lightweight anti-tank weapon which, he told me, would revolutionize battlefield warfare. It could be carried by an infantryman, and it was one shot and throw away, deadly accurate at one kilometre.

I had a look, and the problem was obvious, in that they were using a spray process which mixed the epoxy resin and the hardener, and this was causing an aerosol of highly allergenic epoxy monomer to waft over the whole factory, but was particularly intense immediately adjacent to the workforce.

I explained that the production line needed to be redesigned so that there was a complete seal between the workforce and the spray. Once this had been done there were no more cases of contact dermatitis, and work was able to continue. Shortly afterwards I received a nice letter from the company, with a modest cheque, and a note to explain that but for my intervention, the whole project would have been abandoned because no one had been willing to work at the factory when word had gone round about the skin problems that the workers were experiencing.

I hadn't given this episode much thought for many years. However, in February 2022, Russia initiated what Mr Putin called 'a special military operation' in Ukraine. In the early weeks, it was evident that the bravery and spirit of the Ukrainian resistance were far greater than the Russians had anticipated, and news reports particularly highlighted the role of the British-made NLAW[53] anti-tank weapons, which seemed to be able to bring the convoys of Russian troops to an unexpected halt.

---

53   Next Generation Lightweight Anti-Tank Weapon

My memory suddenly flashed back to my factory visit and the men with their disabling sensitivity to epoxy resin. What they had been working on was one of the earliest prototypes of these guns, which were now being built in Belfast as part of a British-Swedish collaboration, and put to deadly effect.

Sadly, when it seemed that his ground invasion had stalled, Mr Putin resorted to the punitive bombing of civilians. Perhaps without my intervention all those years ago, the war in Ukraine may have had a very different course.

CHAPTER THIRTEEN

ONE LAST ADVENTURE

Mr P was a pleasant man in his early seventies. He had worked hard all his life, building up a successful business, and had always kept himself fit. A few months before I saw him, he had developed a widespread rash, mainly on the sun-exposed parts of his skin, associated with a general feeling of tiredness, shortness of breath and muscle aching.

I diagnosed a condition called lupus, which is an autoimmune disorder in which, for reasons unknown, the immune system starts reacting against the patient's own tissues. He responded well to treatment, although I had to emphasize that it was a long-term condition which needed to be kept under control. At one of his follow-up appointments, he told me that he had booked a holiday. I said that I thought that was an excellent idea, and asked him where he was going.

"Oh, I am taking a 1930s Norton motorbike up the foothills of the Himalayas," he replied.

It wasn't exactly the holiday destination that I had been expecting, and after a few moments of thought, I explained that he ought to think carefully about going somewhere so remote, as there might not be very good medical backup if anything went amiss. I also pointed out that lupus can be aggravated by intense sunlight and that the ultraviolet levels in the Himalayas would be very high.

He came back to see me again a few weeks later. He explained that he had thought about my advice and cancelled the holiday and booked something else. I asked him about his new destination.

"I am going by bicycle over the Pyrenees," he replied.

I hate being a killjoy with my patients, and this was certainly safer than his first plan, but the passes across the Pyrenees are pretty high, and much of the area is quite remote. I told him to take care, use plenty of sun protection, and let me know how he got on.

A little while later, he phoned me up, feeling very despondent. He had gone for a practice cycle in the Lake District, and could only manage forty-five miles. He had cancelled the Pyrenees, as he realised that it was beyond him, and he was still thinking about where he might go. I was beginning to feel more like a travel agent than a doctor and again, said that I thought a nice holiday would still be good for him, as long as he didn't overdo things.

I didn't see him for some months, but when, in due course, he came for a follow-up visit, his lupus seemed in full remission. He was in a cheerful mood. He had booked a holiday which he felt I would approve of, travelling by motorbike from the bottom of South Island in New Zealand to the top of

North Island; nowhere too remote or too mountainous, and everywhere within reach of good healthcare if need be. He was going to be in a group of motorcyclists, and he was sure he could manage it. I wished him well.

It was quite a long time before I saw Mr P again. He was doing well, but when I asked him how the trip to New Zealand had gone, he told me, with a downcast expression, that it had had to be cancelled, as none of his friends could get travel insurance because of a variety of health problems.

More time passed, until one day, out of the blue, he phoned me. He explained that he had finally managed to arrange a trip, had health insurance, and felt all was set, but just wanted to check with me before he set off. He was going to fly to New York, and travel on an old Harley Davidson motorbike from coast to coast, across the United States. I wished him well, and a few weeks later received a postcard from him, postmarked from San Francisco, California. It simply read 'Mission accomplished'. I never heard from him again.

Thinking back about Mr P, I suspect that he had reached an age when he just wanted one last big adventure. I feel pleased that I helped him achieve it.

CHAPTER FOURTEEN

MAGNETIC ATTRACTION

My grandmother was a rather superstitious lady, and when we were growing up, I remember that we were absolutely forbidden ever to discuss anything to do with our health. She firmly believed that if you had never heard of it, you couldn't get it! In retrospect, I think that this was the reason why I was drawn to medicine as a career because the whole subject seemed so shrouded in mystery. It may also explain why I have a tendency to steer well clear of doctors; indeed, until very recently I hadn't consulted a doctor since 2010.

Some months ago, however, I developed an unexplained, persistent, sharp pain just at the tip of my coccyx. I ignored it for about three months, but eventually, I resorted to the Internet, and with a few clicks of the mouse identified a strange ailment called 'coccydynia'. But what might be the cause? I consulted a very helpful NHS website which gave a long list of possibilities, starting with pregnancy and gross obesity, both of which I could quickly exclude. I worked my way through the list until I was left with 'rarely, metastatic malignancy'.

I thought about this for a few minutes and realised that I needed to get some expert advice. But who on earth would be the right person to consult? I asked the outpatient receptionists at my local private hospital who they thought was the best general surgeon, and they all gave the same answer, and an appointment was duly booked.

I wasn't disappointed, as a detailed medical history was taken, and a most thorough, if slightly undignified, physical examination performed, the latter not identifying anything concerning. It was suggested that I had a PSA test[54] (normal) and an MRI scan.

I know little about MRI, it's not something that we often request in dermatology patients, but the helpful radiographers slid me into a tube and gave me some headphones linked to Radio 2, and I lay there trying to let my mind go blank. About halfway through, there was a curious bubbling sensation at exactly the tender point in my coccyx, and all pain instantly vanished, never to be felt again.

In due course, I was phoned with the cheerful news that the MRI was completely normal, but the whole experience set me thinking. I had hitherto imagined that the main purpose of MRI was to reassure neurotic fusspots such as me, but perhaps we are underrating its benefits.

In the nineteenth century, there was a public fascination with the newly discovered effects of electromagnetism. The first device for medical use was built by a Frenchman, Monsieur Hippolyte, in 1832, and subsequently, all sorts of machines, usually housed in rather elegant wooden boxes,

---

54   PSA (prostate-specific antigen) test is a screening test for prostate cancer.

were marketed, promising cures for almost every imaginable ailment. Many claimed remarkable effects on mental disorders, but ladies could purchase electromagnetic corsets to aid weight reduction, and gentlemen were encouraged to use 'Dr Moffat's electromagnetic belt for extra vigour', or 'Dr Scott's electric hairbrush' to combat impending baldness. One could even obtain electromagnetic socks.

These devices, with their elegant brass handles and knobs, now appear from time to time as historic relics on antiques programmes on television, but perhaps from my own experience, we have been premature in abandoning the potential therapeutic effects of magnetism.

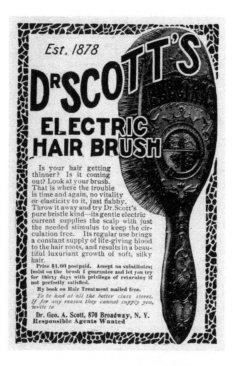

Figure 14: Dr Scott's electric hairbrush (1907)

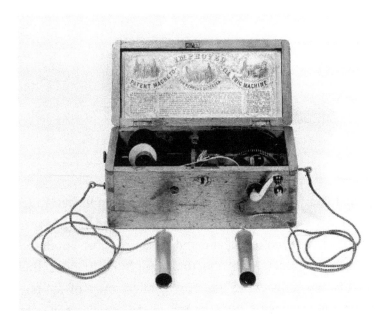

Figure 15: Electrical devices such as this were widely used for a host of medical conditions. No doubt they had a strong placebo effect. (Wellcome Collection)

CHAPTER FIFTEEN

WHAT'S IN A NAME?

Dermatology as a specialty really became established in the latter half of the nineteenth century. At that time, there were few effective treatments, and the cause of most conditions was poorly understood. Doctors had little to offer their patients but a listening ear and gentle words of support. Dermatologists, with little better to do, spent their time describing the appearance of skin disorders in minute detail and thinking up long and difficult names. Any textbook of dermatology is replete with bizarre names such as *mycosis fungoides* and *pityriasis lichenoides*. One of my favourites is *phytophotodermatitis*, not merely for its splendid name, but for the fact that it so frequently causes diagnostic confusion among those who have never seen a case before.

The term phytophotodermatitis was in fact coined in 1942[55], but the condition had been recognised long before that, with a variety of different titles. Essentially the condition occurs when the skin is in contact with the foliage of a number of plants, especially of the parsley or wild turnip families, whose sap contains chemicals called furocoumarins. These chemicals are activated by ultraviolet light and the product of

---

55   R. Klaber, 1942, Phyto-photo-dermatitis. British Journal of Dermatology and Syphilis, Volume 54, 193.

this reaction will cause an irritant burn. In the typical case, a patient will have been weeding an overgrown patch of garden on a sunny day and will present, a few hours later, with painful streaked blisters over the exposed areas of skin.

To the experienced eye, the appearance is characteristic, but to those who are unfamiliar with the condition, misdiagnosis can cause real difficulties. In 1941, a group of soldiers was exercising on Salisbury Plain. It was a warm and sunny day and during their break for lunch, some of them stripped to the waist and lay down to have a rest. The next morning, they were in acute pain, with a blistered rash over their backs. One of the orderlies in the medical centre remembered that something similar had happened to another group of soldiers a couple of years earlier.

The men were admitted to a military hospital for treatment, and rumours soon spread that the area must have been sprayed with toxic nitrogen mustard by the Germans. Fortunately, the Army had the services of an eminent dermatologist, Major William O'Donovan, who aged fifty-seven, had volunteered for medical duties at the outbreak of the War, having previously been the consultant in charge of the dermatology and venereology departments at the London Hospital. O'Donovan was able to reassure everyone that these weren't cases of mustard gas poisoning, but the effects of exposure to the plants which they had been lying on, on a sunny day.

O'Donovan was a larger-than-life character, who had, somewhat improbably, been elected Member of Parliament for the Conservative party in 1930, standing for the Mile End constituency, which served one of the poorest parts of the East End of London and was the area in which his hospital was located. In a subsequent general election, the area elected a Communist, Phil Piriatin, one of only four people ever to be elected as an MP under the Communist banner. [56]

Another curious episode of phytophotodermatitis occurred in the North of England in the 1980s. A group of young offenders on a 'community payback' programme, had been tasked with clearing an overgrown area of banking beside a main road. They had been issued with strimmers to clear the vegetation, and as it was a sunny day, they had all taken off their shirts.

Strimmers work by having a nylon thread which rotates rapidly, and inevitably, little fragments of broken-off vegetation are projected at high speed. By the end of the day, they all had painful red marks in a linear distribution, some of which were beginning to blister, over the abdomen, anterior chest and forearms. The lads demanded that the police were called, claiming that the marks were the result of their supervisors having assaulted them.

They were all taken to a nearby police station and the local police surgeon was summoned. He admitted that the marks looked just like the effect that a whip might have made. Fortunately, he managed to get in contact with a distinguished consultant dermatologist, Dr Adrian Ive[57], who immediately recognised the condition for what it was, a case of

---

56   O'Donovan was also a devout Catholic, and was made a papal knight.
57   For many years he was a consultant in Durham.

phytophotodermatitis, or as he cheerfully labelled it 'strimmer dermatitis'. At the time, garden strimmers were quite new, but it is now a story with which every dermatologist is familiar, and the name 'strimmer dermatitis' has stuck.

I see cases of phytophotodermatitis quite regularly, almost always on a Monday morning in early summer, after a sunny weekend. The call is usually from an anxious doctor in Accident and Emergency, and on several occasions, when a child has been the victim, presenting with a livid blistering rash, the possibility of child abuse has been suggested.

Once you have managed to elicit the history of the child having been playing in overgrown vegetation and the linear nature of the blistering demonstrated, the diagnosis becomes obvious. It is always lovely being able to reassure everyone that the parents are blameless, and to tell the parents that the rash will get better in a few days.

CHAPTER SIXTEEN

TIMES HAVE CHANGED

When I started as a consultant in 1987, we all had lunch in the consultants' dining room. This wasn't anywhere smart; indeed, the furnishings were rather shabby, and food was fairly basic, except on Fridays when we were served fish and chips. It was a facility which didn't cost the hospital any money, as we paid for what we ate. Most importantly, it was a short break in the middle of the day when important business was discussed. We got to know each other, and face to face it was easy to resolve clinical problems or to discuss organisational issues in the hospital.

Most importantly, our local GP colleagues often popped in to join us. We got to know them, and they often asked for advice about patients. The cordial relations between the GPs and consultants created an atmosphere where there was no sense of 'us and them'; we worked as a single team to the benefit of our patients.

One of those GPs who I remember well from my early years as a consultant was Dr W. He had qualified in medicine in 1938, and joined the Royal Army Medical Corps at the outbreak of the War. He had been posted to the Far East, was captured by the Japanese at the fall of Singapore and spent four years as a prisoner of war, on the notorious Burma railway. On his return, he took over a single-handed practice in a rural part of our county which had previously been run by his father.

Even in the 1980s, the practice had been run in an eccentric fashion. There was no appointment system, nor any computer-based records, and patients queued outside his house, before being ushered into his front room where consultations took place. Requests for repeat prescriptions had to be pinned to a noticeboard at the local petrol station, from where the completed prescriptions could be collected the next day. In those distant days, before any of us had heard of 'data protection', there was nothing to prevent people from having a quick look at their neighbours' prescriptions, and gossiping about what might be wrong with them.

His referral letters were short and to the point. He often simply wrote 'rash', in which case you could be certain that the patient had a nasty rash requiring urgent attention. Sometimes he wrote 'rash?'. 'Rash?' was quite different from simply 'rash', as it meant that the patient said that they had a rash, but that he hadn't actually examined them.

On one memorable occasion, I received a referral which simply said 'penis?'. I was intrigued. When the patient arrived, he was an elderly man, accompanied by an unpleasant odour. When he undressed to be examined, I really couldn't work out what was going on in his lower regions; the label 'penis?' was quite correct.

I called in my colleague, the late Dr Brian Drake, our venereology specialist, who was consulting in an adjacent room, and he was as puzzled as I was. He asked the patient when he had last had sexual intercourse, to which he replied, "The night of the Queen's coronation, 1953." In the circumstances, we agreed that it was unlikely to be a sexually transmitted disease.

Eventually, one of my surgical colleagues and I arranged to examine the affected area under general anaesthetic, and a biopsy was taken which showed that the poor chap had an advanced and neglected cancer of the penis, from which he subsequently died. The GP's referral with 'Penis?' was right on the mark.

Dr W consulted me himself on one occasion. As a prisoner of war, he had acquired a fungal infection of his finger and toenails. At the time, this was something which was very difficult to treat, until, in 1959, a new antifungal drug, griseofulvin, became available.[58] Unfortunately, Dr W was allergic to griseofulvin, and for many years his unsightly, crumbling nails had been a constant reminder of the horrors of his captivity.

Purely by chance, just at the time that he came to see me, a new, safer antifungal drug, terbinafine, had just been launched, and I started him on treatment. It proved remarkably effective in his case, and I have rarely encountered a more grateful patient.

---

58   See Chapter 10, 'Keep Your Hair On'

A little while later, I heard that, rather late in life, he had met and married a Jewish lady who had survived captivity in a Nazi concentration camp. Perhaps my treatment had played a small part in him finally conquering his demons and finding happiness.

When he died, he was deeply mourned by his patients and is still fondly remembered by many of them. It was a different way of practising medicine, but it seemed to work.

CHAPTER SEVENTEEN

AN ITCHY BUSINESS

Dr J was a well-known local GP, popular and well-regarded by both his patients and his medical colleagues, so I was very flattered when he asked whether he could come and see me as a patient.

He explained that he had suffered from the most intractable itching of his skin for several years, and it had come to torment him. His sleep was disturbed and he kept his wife awake with his restlessness and nocturnal scratching, and in the morning his sheets were covered in blood. He was otherwise fit and well, and blood tests performed by his own GP were entirely normal. He had tried all manner of creams and ointments, added all sorts of preparations to his bath, and taken endless courses of antibiotics and other possible remedies, all to no avail. He had even resorted to alternative medicines and hypnosis, but nothing had helped.

"I don't suppose that there's anything you can do," he added, "but I am at my wit's end."

What do you do in this sort of situation? The answer is obvious, in that you need to start from the beginning with a careful history and a full examination of the skin.

It seemed that the itching started with clusters of tiny blisters that provoked intense scratching so that the skin was soon broken. These arose especially on the scalp, backs of the shoulders, lower back and buttocks, elbows and knees. The scratching, of course, left its own marks and sometimes bleeding or secondary bacterial infection.

After I had examined him, I said, "Well, I think I know what the problem is." He looked at me with a somewhat mystified expression. "This all looks very much like dermatitis herpetiformis."

Dermatitis herpetiformis is a strange condition, which often leads to diagnostic confusion. Despite the name, it has nothing to do with 'herpes', herpetiformis means 'looking like herpes', in that there are little clusters of blisters, as occur in a herpetic cold sore. However, it is not caused by a virus but is an autoimmune disorder, in which the patient's immune system produces antibodies which react against the skin. It is associated with gluten sensitivity, although many patients have no symptoms relating to the digestive system.

I explained to him that we needed to do a biopsy to confirm the diagnosis, as the laboratory is able to demonstrate the deposition of autoantibodies in the skin by a rather clever method called direct immunofluorescence. I also suggested to him that while we were waiting for the result of the biopsy, which might take a couple of weeks, we could give him a clinical trial with a drug called dapsone.

Dapsone is a very curious drug. The molecule was initially synthesised in the first decade of the twentieth century, but it was over thirty years before it was realised that it had any clinical application. However, over the years, it has come to be used in a number of different conditions, including leprosy, malaria, acne, and various rheumatological conditions.[59] To this day, no one really understands quite how it works.

At the beginning of the Second World War, both the British and the Germans, aware of the horrific toll of battlefield injuries in the First World War, were keen to find an effective antibacterial drug. Although the discovery of penicillin is associated with the name of Alexander Fleming, it was Florey and Chain and their team, at Oxford, who realised its importance and demonstrated its efficacy.[60] Subsequent mass production of the drug saved the lives of countless wounded soldiers, but penicillin also had an important effect on military morale; soldiers were assured that even if they were injured, effective treatment would be available.

The Germans also put considerable effort into investigating antibacterials, and one of the agents that they looked at was diaminodiphenyl sulphone (dapsone). Horrific experiments were conducted on inmates of Buchenwald concentration camp, to see whether dapsone reduced the subsequent development of bacterial infection in chemical burns of the

---

59   Its use in leprosy was discovered in the 1950s, and it is still part of the standard treatment. The effect of dapsone in malaria was discovered by the US military during the Vietnam War.

60   Fleming never appreciated the significance of his own discovery, although he was happy to take much of the credit. Fleming, Florey and Chain shared the Nobel Prize for Medicine in 1945.

skin. Dapsone was shown to have some mild anti-bacterial and anti-inflammatory effect, but appeared to have little clinical application.

One observation that was made was that if the dose of dapsone was too high, the prisoners became acutely unwell, with severe shortness of breath and cyanosis.[61] Quite a few of them died. This was due to the development of methaemoglobinaemia. Oxygen is normally carried around the body attached to haemoglobin in the red blood cells. Each molecule of haemoglobin has an iron atom, and the iron is in the ferrous state. Dapsone can convert the iron to the ferric state, methaemoglobin, which cannot transport oxygen.

I have only once seen a case of methaemoglobinaemia when I was a medical registrar at Westminster Hospital and had never even heard of the condition. Fortunately, my consultant, Dr Richard Staughton, recognised the problem. The antidote is a dye called methylene blue, and I was told to run down to the pharmacy to obtain an ampoule of it, which I was instructed to inject intravenously. Almost like a conjuring trick, the patient immediately turned a healthy pink colour, but for the next twenty-four hours, they passed bright blue urine, as the methylene blue was excreted.

The effect of dapsone in dermatitis herpetiformis was discovered largely by chance in the early 1950s, and it certainly is dramatic. Two days after I prescribed it for Dr J, he phoned me to say that he had slept through the night without being

---

61   Blueness of the extremities, lips and tongue.

kept awake by itching for the first time in ten years. The rash was already fading.

In case anyone reading this is tempted to try dapsone for an itchy skin condition, I should say that its effect is quite specific for dermatitis herpetiformis, and it has no effect at all on other itchy skin conditions such as eczema and urticaria.

Once I had received confirmation of the diagnosis from the laboratory, I started Dr J on a gluten-free diet, which is an important part of the treatment, and he does have to remain on a small dose of dapsone. Even after many years, if he misses a dose for more than a day, the condition comes back until he restarts it. It is a small price to pay to be free of itching.

One of his children became a doctor and is now a consultant dermatologist. I have never asked whether their father's miraculous cure influenced their career choice.

CHAPTER EIGHTEEN

A HISTORY LESSON

Taking a proper medical history is the most important part of any consultation; you never quite know what the patient is going to tell you.

Mr R was seventy and had been referred by his GP with a lump on his shoulder which had appeared over the preceding three months and which the GP was suspicious of being a type of skin cancer. It was now about three centimetres in diameter, had an ulcerated surface and a tendency to bleed. The appearance and the history were very suggestive of a potentially serious type of skin cancer called a squamous cell carcinoma.

Going through the medical history, I asked whether he was on any medications, and he explained that he was on quite a cocktail of immunosuppressive drugs. This was potentially most significant, because patients who are immunosuppressed, for whatever reason, have a greatly increased risk of skin cancer, and those cancers can run a much more aggressive course. I inquired why he was on these drugs, and he explained that five years previously he had undergone a liver transplant. In such patients, immunosuppression is essential to prevent the rejection of the transplanted organ.

Organ transplantation is one of the medical miracles of the last fifty years. Because of their risk of developing skin cancers, we see quite a lot of transplant patients in a dermatology clinic, and they never cease to amaze me. I vividly remember seeing a man in my clinic who told me that he had had a heart transplant several years previously. As I looked at him, I suddenly realised that I had met him before; he was a builder, and a few months earlier had been climbing up and down a ladder while doing some repairs to the roof of my house. It was extraordinary to think that someone who had been at death's door with heart failure could be restored to such robust fitness.

Mr R also looked remarkably well, and I asked him why he had needed a transplant. He explained that he had developed a form of liver cancer called hepatoma. Hepatoma usually arises in patients who have pre-existing severe liver disease, most commonly chronic infection with Hepatitis C, which was, in fact, the cause in Mr R's case. I was a bit puzzled, as Hepatitis C is most commonly seen in intravenous drug users, and I didn't think that he was quite the type. I was also rather concerned, as patients with Hepatitis C are potentially highly infectious if you operate on them, and it seemed I would be having to remove his skin cancer.

I carried on unravelling his history and asked how it was thought that he had acquired Hepatitis C. He explained that he had haemophilia, and he was likely to have been infected in the 1980s as a result of his treatment. His original diagnosis had been made when he was nine and had a dental extraction, which resulted in severe bleeding requiring blood transfusions.

Haemophilia is an inherited disorder of blood clotting. Severe bleeding may occur after minor injuries, or, for example, dental extractions as in my patient's case. One particular problem is spontaneous, painful bleeding into joints, which often only heal with severe deformity.

Haemophilia is inherited on the female side, but only produces symptoms in the males. Historians believe that Queen Victoria was a carrier of the disorder, as several members of the European royal families, all of whom were interrelated, were affected.[62] At one time it was commonly referred to as 'the royal disease'. One of those who was affected was Alexei, the young son of Czar Nicolas II of Russia. A man called Grigori Rasputin, who was something of a charlatan, convinced the Czar and his wife that he had mystical powers which could cure Alexei. Rasputin acquired considerable influence at Court, and there are those that believe that his malign influence played a significant part in sowing the seeds of discontent that led to the 1917 Russian Revolution.

We now know that haemophilia is caused by a deficiency of Factor VIII, one of the elements of the clotting pathway.[63] The first effective treatment was with concentrates of blood

---

62   There is a good account of this by Richard Stevens, The history of haemophilia in the royal families of Europe, British Journal of Haematology, 2005, volume 105, 25-32

63   In fact, in a small proportion of cases the defect is in Factor IX; this is called haemophilia B, often termed Christmas Disease. The name has nothing to do with December 25th, but was the surname of the first patient to be diagnosed with the condition. It is the only disease that I know of which is named after a patient; most, of course are named after the person who discovered it, or occasionally, as in Lyme disease, the place where it was first identified.

plasma, which could be given by injection for episodes of bleeding, or as a preventative if the patient needed an operation or dental extraction.

In the UK, a network of fifty hospitals which held stocks of plasma concentrate was established, and patients were given a list so they knew where they could get help. One of the hospitals was in Bournemouth, where I worked for a year as a medical registrar in 1978. It became a popular choice of holiday resort for patients with haemophilia. I never ceased to be amazed by the recklessness of many of these patients, who seemed to spend their whole vacation diving off rocks or falling off cliffs, before having to rush for an emergency injection.

Unfortunately, the product that was used, imported from the United States, was a concentrate of clotting factors; extracted blood taken from donors and pooled, and a single dose may have had material from many thousands of individual donors. At that time, we were less aware than we are today of the risk of transmitting blood-borne viruses and it is now known that over four thousand patients in the UK with haemophilia and other clotting disorders were infected with HIV or Hepatitis C from the imported pooled plasma concentrate. The majority of those patients died, and it was only by chance that my patient had avoided being infected with HIV as well. It is terrible to think that it is likely that many of those carefree holidaymakers who I helped to treat were among those who were victims.[64]

---

64 Nowadays, haemophilia can be treated with an entirely synthetic form of genetically engineered Factor VIII, without no risk to the patient of viral transmission.

Now that I understood the sequence of events, I was still left with a problem. My patient needed an operation to remove his skin cancer, but he had haemophilia and was potentially at risk of severe bleeding, and he had Hepatitis C so that meant I was at significant risk in performing the surgery.

I explained the situation to Mr R.

"Oh, don't worry," he reassured me, "the transplant has cured my haemophilia."

I was still puzzled. How could he have been cured of a genetic disease? But in fact, he was right, because Factor VIII, the missing clotting factor, is normally synthesised in the liver, and there are now a number of patients who have been cured by liver transplantation. With regard to the Hepatitis C, he was also able to update my medical knowledge. In the last few years, new anti-viral drugs have been developed which effectively eliminate Hepatitis C virus from the system, and he had been treated prior to his transplant to ensure that his new liver was not infected and that he was no longer infectious.

His skin cancer was treated uneventfully, without excessive bleeding and without me catching hepatitis, but if I hadn't taken a proper medical history, I would never have heard his extraordinary tale. And I also learned how much we depend on patients to keep our medical knowledge up to date, and how important it is to listen to them.

As a postscript, in 2019 an independent public inquiry into the effects of infected blood products began to take evidence and made its preliminary report in 2022.[65] Among those who gave evidence were relatives of people who had died, and a number of survivors, including my patient. The government has agreed on a package of compensation for the ever-diminishing number of survivors, but sadly, for most of those affected, it is too late.

---

65   Details can be read on www.infectedbloodinquiry.org.uk

CHAPTER NINETEEN

SHEFFIELD STEEL

Sometimes objects which we handle every day seem so unremarkable that we don't give them a moment's thought. Although dermatology is a 'medical' specialty, we do quite a lot of skin surgery, excising skin cancers, taking diagnostic biopsies and so on. One day, I was just about to perform a fairly routine procedure when I started to look at the packaging of the surgical blade. So much British manufacturing industry has vanished over the years that I was rather surprised to see that the blade was made in England.

In fact, it turns out that Swann-Morton blades, made by WR Swann and Co Ltd, are not just used in virtually every operation performed in the NHS, but are exported all over the world, and they are still made exclusively in Sheffield, the traditional home of blade-making. Not only has the company 'bucked the trend' but it has a rather remarkable history, almost certainly unknown to most of those that use its products.

Walter Robinson Swann was born in Sheffield in 1900. He won a scholarship to Sheffield Grammar School, and aged sixteen entered work in the steel trade. Since the seventeenth century, Sheffield had been renowned the world over for steel making and for the manufacture of fine steel products. It was often called 'steel city', one of the local football teams, Sheffield United, are still called 'the blades' by their fans, and the London to Sheffield express train was called 'The Master Cutler'. In the centre of Sheffield, there is a magnificent building called Cutlers' Hall, the headquarters of the Worshipful Company of Cutlers, which contains a magnificent collection of locally made metalwork.

Walter Swann was an idealistic young man and horrified by the working conditions that many of the factory workers had to endure. In 1917, news came of the Russian Revolution, and Swann was fascinated. He dreamed of the idea of the Sheffield steel industry being run on revolutionary socialist principles, not something that endeared him to his employers.

By 1932, he had saved a small amount of capital, and together with a friend, JA Morton, a metallurgist, opened his own company, and right from the start was determined to apply his socialist business ideas. Initially, they manufactured razor blades, and the early adverts stated that the blades had been made in a 'forty-hour week factory', a clear distinction from the long hours that his competitors required of their staff. As business thrived, he bought a small fruit farm in Cambridgeshire and arranged for supplies of fresh fruit to be sent to his workers.

His real breakthrough came in 1935 when he switched to making surgical blades. The two-part scalpel, with a disposable blade detachable from the handle had been invented in 1915 by an American, Morgan Parker, who had gone into partnership with a medical equipment supplier, Charles Bard, to form the Bard-Parker company. However, in 1935, Bard and Parker had fallen out and somehow had failed to renew their patent.[66] Walter Swann took his opportunity, and by the early 1950s, they were the market leader in surgical blades. They subsequently became the first company to use gamma radiation to sterilize blades.

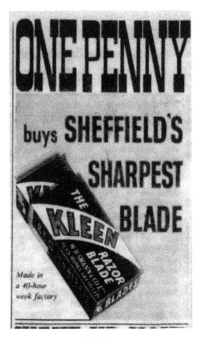

Figure 16: Early advert from WR Swann and Co Ltd. Note the 'Made in a 40-hour week factory'. By permission of Grace's Guide.

As the company grew, Walter Swann worried about what would happen as he got older, and in 1960 he transferred

---

66   Bard-Parker, subsequently re-named Bard, became one of the largest medical devices companies in the world, but came to a sticky end after a number of high-profile legal cases relating to allegedly faulty products.

ownership to an employees' trust. The employees became the owners, and each year the profits are shared, half going to the workforce, and half being given to medical charities, mainly local hospitals in Sheffield and the Royal College of Surgeons.

On his first day at work in his new business, Walter Swann placed a hand-written note on the door, stating the principles on which the company was to run. The note is still, carefully preserved, on show at the company's head office, and one of his statements reads 'If the management cannot do the job, a new management is required.' Perhaps that is something that the NHS should reflect upon.

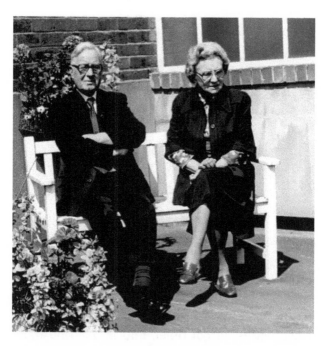

Figure 17: Walter Swann with his long-time factory manager
Doris Fairweather outside their factory
(by Permission of WR Swann and Co Ltd).

CHAPTER TWENTY

LAST WORDS

I was sitting at home, just making the final corrections to the manuscript of this book, prior to sending it off to the editor, when the postman pushed a pile of letters through my letter box. There was the usual selection of adverts, circulars, and bills, but amongst them was a letter from one of my colleagues, a consultant ENT surgeon.

It began, "Dear Barry, I saw Mr X in my clinic, and I wonder whether you remember him from when you saw him in 2007? He is still doing well, and asked to be remembered to you."

I certainly did remember Mr X, although I hadn't seen him for some fifteen years, and his was one of those cases which reminds you why a career in medicine is so satisfying, and his story just couldn't be left out of this book.

Mr X was in his fifties when he presented to the ENT department, with a story of having 'blocked ears' for about six months. He had seen my colleague who had been very puzzled. As he explained to me, the appearance of skin in the ears was unusual, and there was bleeding with the slightest touch of the otoscope. "Would you please see him, and see if there was any dermatological explanation?"

I saw him a couple of weeks later, and he told me that in addition to the problem with his ears, he had been feeling generally unwell, and had been under the cardiology department with low blood pressure, an irregular pulse and an enlarged heart, for which there was, as yet, no explanation.

Looking at him, as I listened to his story, the most striking thing was the appearance of his face, with spectacular bruising of his eyelids and around his eyes, which made him look something like a panda; he explained that this appeared whenever he had a bout of coughing.

When I came to examine him, I noted that he had an exceptionally large tongue, and when I commented on this, he said that he had noticed recently that he had been accidentally biting his tongue when he chewed his food. He also mentioned that he had recently noticed bruising and skin fragility of his penis when he attempted sexual intercourse.

The story of skin fragility, bruising around the eyes ('panda eyes'), and enlargement of the tongue ('macroglossia') are absolutely typical of a very rare disorder known as systemic amyloidosis. Although rare, it is one of those disorders which if you have ever seen it, you will recognise it at once.

Amyloidosis is a disorder in which a protein called amyloid is deposited in the tissues of various organs. In the skin, it is deposited around blood vessels and results in bleeding into the skin and general fragility, so that blistering readily occurs. The diagnosis is most reliably confirmed by taking a small specimen of fat from under the surface of the skin of the abdomen, and asking the pathology laboratory to stain the sample with a dye 'Congo red'; examination under the microscope reveals a beautiful apple green colour when viewed with polarized light.

I have only seen a handful of cases of primary amyloidosis over the years, and when I first started in dermatology it was a dreadful diagnosis to make. No effective treatment was available, and the interval between diagnosis and death was usually about twelve months. One felt like a judge putting on his black cap to pronounce the sentence in a murder case in the days of capital punishment.

Fortunately for Mr X, by 2007, it was being recognised that systemic amyloidosis was caused by an abnormal clone of malignant cells in the bone marrow which produce the amyloid protein, and that targeted treatment was highly effective.

I referred him to the Royal Free Hospital in London, where they have a national service for patients with amyloidosis. A scan showed amyloid deposits in his heart, which probably explained his heart problems, as well as in his skin and his tongue but not elsewhere. This was fortunate, as amyloid deposition in the kidneys can cause renal failure, and deposition in the peripheral nervous system may cause severe neuropathy. Systemic treatment has controlled the underlying bone marrow disorder. He remains under their care, and fifteen years on lives a full and active life.

For all the tribulations of our everyday working lives as doctors, cases like this are what make it all worthwhile, and also shows the immeasurable value of long-term follow-up and continuity of care.

ACKNOWLEDGEMENTS

It has been an immense privilege to have been a doctor for over forty years, and every day still brings surprises. I am grateful to all of my patients over the years who have put their trust in me and from whom I have learned so much. I must also mention, with eternal thanks, those who helped me on my way, especially Dr Richard Staughton, who first inspired me to pursue dermatology as a career, and the late Dr Imrich Sarkany, who gave me my first job as a registrar at the Royal Free, and Dr Anthony du Vivier and Dr Andrew Pembroke, at King's College Hospital, from whom I learned so much.

My uncle, Professor Harold Ellis, has been a mentor and guide throughout my career, and this book wouldn't have been written without his encouragement and guidance.

I am once again most grateful to the team at *Spiffing Covers* for helping turn a manuscript into the finished article. My friend, Jill Stephen, also helped with sorting out my grammar and punctuation and with general encouragement.

At work, I am supported by a wonderful team, Hilary, Linsay, and Hazel, who keep the show on the road, and do their best to keep me out of trouble. Work can be hectic, but they always make it fun.

At home, Margaret has a special place in my heart, encourages and supports me, and makes it all worthwhile.

ABOUT THE AUTHOR

Dr Barry Monk studied medicine at Jesus College, Cambridge, and Westminster Medical School, qualifying as a doctor in 1975. After junior hospital posts in London, Cambridge and Bournemouth, he trained in dermatology at the Royal Free and King's College hospitals. He was appointed a consultant dermatologist in 1987 and finally retired from the NHS in January 2020. He continues to undertake expert medicolegal work in medical negligence cases and private practice in dermatology. In 2008, he served as President of the Section of Dermatology of the Royal Society of Medicine. His previous book, Lifeline, won the British Medical Association 2022 medical books award in the category: 'Good Medical Practice.'

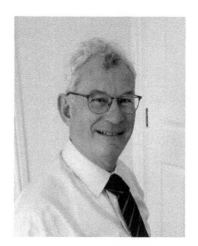

Ingram Content Group UK Ltd.
Milton Keynes UK
UKHW011306100323
418378UK00004B/281